100 QUESTIONS & ANSWERS

ABOUT
Muscular Dystrophy

Kathryn R. Wagner, MD, PhD

Director, Center for Genetic Muscle Disorders
Kennedy Krieger Institute
and
Professor of Neurology and Neuroscience
Johns Hopkins School of Medicine

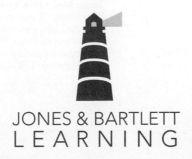

JONES & BARTLETT
LEARNING

World Headquarters
Jones & Bartlett Learning
5 Wall Street
Burlington, MA 01803
978-443-5000
info@jblearning.com
www.jblearning.com

Jones & Bartlett Learning books and products are available through most bookstores and online booksellers. To contact Jones & Bartlett Learning directly, call 800-832-0034, fax 978-443-8000, or visit our website, www.jblearning.com.

Substantial discounts on bulk quantities of Jones & Bartlett Learning publications are available to corporations, professional associations, and other qualified organizations. For details and specific discount information, contact the special sales department at Jones & Bartlett Learning via the above contact information or send an email to specialsales@jblearning.com.

Production Credits
Director of Product Management: Amanda Martin
Product Manager: Joanna Gallant
Product Assistant: Melina Leon
Project Specialist: Dan Stone
Marketing Manager: Lindsay White
Product Fulfillment Manager: Wendy Kilborn
Composition: S4Carlisle Publishing Services
Cover Design: Scott Moden
Rights & Permissions Manager: John Rusk
Senior Media Development Editor: Troy Liston
Cover Image: Courtesy of Levi Gershkowitz, Living in the Light - www.FromPatientToPerson.com; Courtesy of Tayjus Surampudi
Printing and Binding: LSC Communications
Cover Printing: LSC Communications

ISBN: 978-1-284-20166-6

6048

Printed in the United States of America
24 23 22 21 20   10 9 8 7 6 5 4 3 2 1

Dedication

To Kaley Kathryn Vides, who every day shows us how to live with courage, perseverance, and authenticity.

CONTENTS

Contents

Preface   ix

Part One: The Basics   1

Questions 1–6 discuss fundamental questions patients and caregivers have about muscular dystrophy, including:

1. What is muscular dystrophy?
2. What are the initial signs of muscular dystrophy?
3. How is muscular dystrophy diagnosed?
4. How do I find good medical care?
5. What should I expect at a neurology appointment?
6. How can I connect with other families affected with muscular dystrophy?

Part Two: Genetics   19

Questions 7–14 give information about the genetic underpinnings of muscular dystrophy, including:

7. How did I get this disease?
8. Should I have genetic testing?
9. What kinds of genetic testing are available?
10. What is exome sequencing?
11. Can I pass muscular dystrophy on to my children?
12. Should my child have genetic testing?
13. How do I tell my child that he or she has muscular dystrophy?
14. How can I find a genetic counselor?

Part Three: Keeping Muscles Strong   43

Questions 15–24 describe muscle weakness and ways to maintain muscle strength, including:

15. Why are my muscles weak?
16. How weak will I get?
17. Is it safe to exercise?
18. What are the goals of physical therapy?
19. What is occupational therapy?
20. Are supplements for muscles effective and safe to take?

21. Do corticosteroids help?
22. Does testosterone make muscle stronger?
23. What about bracing?
24. What are some general rules regarding stretching?

Part Four: New Therapeutic Options   67

Questions 25–32 describe recent therapeutic advances for muscular
   dystrophy:

25. What is exon skipping?
26. What is gene therapy?
27. What is genome editing?
28. What are stem cells?
29. What is a clinical trial?
30. How do I find a clinical trial in which to participate?
31. How do I qualify for a clinical trial?
32. What's involved in a muscle biopsy?

Part Five: Breathing   85

Questions 33–41 discuss strategies for maintaining respiratory health in muscular
   dystrophy, including:

33. Should I get the influenza vaccine and other recommended vaccines?
34. What is spirometry?
35. What is cough assist?
36. When should I start using nighttime ventilatory support?
37. What's the difference between BIPAP and CPAP?
38. What are the advantages and disadvantages of noninvasive mechanical
    ventilation?
39. What is a sip and puff ventilator?
40. What are the advantages and disadvantages of invasive
    mechanical ventilation?
41. What are some things to remember when going to the emergency
    department?

Part Six: The Heart   101

Questions 42–47 describe effects of muscular dystrophy on the heart and how to
   maintain cardiac health:

42. Why do I need an electrocardiogram?
43. What is an echocardiogram?
44. How can I protect my heart?
45. What is a pacemaker?
46. What is an implantable cardioverter defibrillator?
47. What are advance directives?

Part Seven: Eating and Nutrition   *115*

Questions 48–53 provide information patients and caregivers need about nutrition, including:

48. What are some nutritional recommendations?
49. What is a healthy weight?
50. Does alcohol affect muscles?
51. What's involved in a swallowing study?
52. What is a gastrostomy tube?
53. Is constipation a symptom of muscular dystrophy?

Part Eight: Bone Health   *129*

Questions 54–57 provide recommendations for maintaining bone health in muscular dystrophy:

54. What is a DEXA scan?
55. How can I improve my bone density?
56. How much vitamin D should I take?
57. I've had a fracture—now what?

Part Nine: Mental Health   *139*

Questions 58–63 examine mental health issues in muscular dystrophy, such as:

58. What should I do if I'm depressed or anxious?
59. What is the purpose of a neuropsychological evaluation?
60. Are there support groups?
61. What is executive dysfunction?
62. What is obsessive–compulsive disorder?
63. Would a service animal be helpful?

Part Ten: Pain and Fatigue   *155*

Questions 64–67 explain how pain and fatigue are addressed in muscular dystrophy:

64. How can I treat my pain?
65. What can I do about fatigue?
66. Should I push through my pain and fatigue to increase strength and stamina?
67. What is palliative care?

Part Eleven: Surgeries   *165*

Questions 68–72 discuss surgical procedures patients may elect to treat symptoms of muscular dystrophy, including:

68. When is scoliosis surgery recommended?
69. Should I get tendon releases?

70. Who could benefit from scapular fixation?
71. What is ptosis repair?
72. What precautions should be taken with anesthesia?

Part Twelve: School and Muscular Dystrophy   *175*

Questions 73–80 discuss issues patients encounter related to school:
73. When should I tell the school about the diagnosis?
74. What are IEP and 504 plans?
75. Which is a better option—private or public school?
76. What is a paraprofessional?
77. What are reasonable accommodations that a school should make?
78. What help is there for reading and writing?
79. What are treatment options for attention deficit hyperactivity disorder?
80. How does one prepare a child with muscular dystrophy for college?

Part Thirteen: Work and Muscular Dystrophy   *201*

Questions 81–86 discuss issues related to working with muscular dystrophy:
81. When and what should I share with my employer?
82. What are reasonable accommodations that a workplace should make?
83. Should I keep working?
84. What are disability benefits?
85. What is the Family Medical Leave Act?
86. How do I get personal care attendant support?

Part Fourteen: Play and Muscular Dystrophy   *217*

Questions 87–90 discuss issues related to playing sports, playing games, and traveling with muscular dystrophy:
87. What are adaptive sports?
88. What options are there for a computer mouse or controller?
89. What are appropriate limits for video games and online socialization?
90. What are some tips for airplane travel?

Part Fifteen: Sexual Health Issues   *229*

Questions 91–92 discuss issues related to sexual relationships and muscular dystrophy:
91. What about dating and sex?
92. What if I want to get pregnant?

Part Sixteen: Assistive Equipment 235

Questions 93–100 describe assistive equipment that may be useful for patients with muscular dystrophy:

93. Should I get a scooter or a wheelchair?
94. What features should I look for in a wheelchair?
95. What is a stander?
96. When should I get a hospital bed?
97. What equipment options are there for bathing?
98. What help is there for transfers?
99. What is a loan closet?
100. Can I drive?

Appendix A: Abbreviations 257

*Appendix B: Foundations That Support Patients
and/or Research* 259

Glossary 261

Index 267

Acknowledgments 276

PREFACE

Preface

Muscular dystrophies (MDs) are rare disorders. However, collectively, there are an estimated 250,000 individuals in the United States with one of these disorders. Those affected by muscular dystrophy (MD), including patients and families, have many questions, some of which are best answered by healthcare providers, others by those living in the trenches. This book addresses many of the most common questions.

To answer these questions, I drew upon my 20 years of experience caring for those with MD at the Johns Hopkins School of Medicine and Kennedy Krieger Institute. My patients have been the richest source of the information that I'll now share with you. Numerous individuals had input into this book. Four are quoted in these pages: Tayjus, a college-educated young man with Duchenne MD (DMD); Vicky, a mother of a teenager with DMD; Lilleen, a businesswoman with facioscapulohumeral MD (FSHD) and also a mother of a son with FSHD; and Colin, an active sailor with myotonic MD (DM). Each gives an important and different perspective to the questions.

There are over 50 different types of MDs. They differ in the ways they are inherited, in which muscles are affected, in the age of onset, and in what other body systems are involved. For example, some MDs affect heart muscle and others do not. Consequently, not all chapters will apply to every reader, and it is not necessary that you read this book front to back. I hope that you will turn to the questions that most interest you.

I am often asked why I focus my clinical practice and research on MD. The simple answer is that my patients inspire and motivate me. Those living with MD soldier on despite serious challenges. They are not defined by their disease. This book aims to reduce one of the challenges—the gathering of crucial information—by providing it here in an easily accessible format.

Kathryn R. Wagner, MD, PhD

PART ONE

The Basics

What is muscular dystrophy?

What are the initial signs of muscular dystrophy?

How is muscular dystrophy diagnosed?

More . . .

1. What is muscular dystrophy?

Muscular dystrophy (MD) is defined as being a genetic and **progressive** disorder of muscle. This differentiates it from acquired, progressive disorders of muscle such as myositis (an autoimmune disorder) and from genetic, nonprogressive myopathies termed congenital myopathies. With a few exceptions, muscular dystrophies (MDs) are marked by degeneration of muscle fibers, the cells that make up the bulk of the muscle body. These muscle fibers are replaced over time with fat and **fibrosis** (scar tissue). This replacement leads to progressive muscle weakness.

There are over 50 different types of MD. The most common forms are Duchenne muscular dystrophy (DMD), myotonic muscular dystrophy (two forms: DM1 and DM2), and facioscapulohumeral muscular dystrophy (two forms: FSHD1 and FSHD2). There are also many less common forms of MD, including Becker muscular dystrophy (BMD), congenital muscular dystrophy (CMD), Emery-Dreifus muscular dystrophy (EDMD), and oculopharyngeal muscular dystrophy (OPMD). Limb-girdle muscular dystrophy (LGMD) and distal muscular dystrophy (DD) refer to groups of diseases that affect the shoulders and hips (LGMD) or the forearms, hands, lower legs, and feet (distal muscular dystrophy [DD]).

In general, the MDs are due to mutations in different genes. Exceptions are DMD and BMD, which are both due to mutations in the gene for dystrophin and are thus said to be **allelic disorders**. Because of this difference in the genetic cause of the disease, the MDs have unique appearances. For example, some affect the muscles of the face (FSHD, DM, OPMD) while in others,

Progressive

A condition that gradually worsens over time.

Fibrosis

The condition in which muscle in MD is replaced over time with scar tissue in addition to fat.

Allelic disorders

Two or more distinct conditions caused by changes or variants in the same gene.

these muscles are spared. Each MD has a specific pattern of muscles that are affected, although sometimes these patterns overlap, as is the case for many of the LGMDs.

MDs can affect other organs such as the brain, eye, heart, and gastrointestinal tract. Whether or not your other organs will be affected depends on what type of MD you have. Some MDs affect only the muscles of the trunk and limbs. Others affect a wide variety of organ systems. Your neurologist and genetics counselor should inform you about what other systems may be affected in your disease and refer you to the relevant specialists.

2. What are the initial signs of muscular dystrophy?

The initial sign of MD is almost always weakness. The time of life at which this starts (childhood, adolescence, or adulthood) varies depending on the specific MD. Some MDs typically begin in childhood (e.g., DMD, EDMD, CMD). Others typically begin in adulthood (e.g., OPMD, DD). Still others can begin either in childhood *or* adulthood (BMD, FSHD, DM, LGMD). Which muscles are first affected varies across the MDs.

In CMD, early onset FSHD, and congenital DM1, the initial signs of MD occur in infancy. The infant may have poor muscle tone and be described as "floppy." He or she may have difficulty holding up the head when lifted by the arms. Feeding may be difficult due to a weak suck. Occasionally, the infant has difficulty breathing independently.

Children with MD frequently have a delay in their developmental motor milestones. **Developmental delay** refers to a condition in which a child is not developing or achieving skills according to the expected time frame. Your pediatrician should ask you about your child's development at each well-child visit. Children with MD may be late walkers or toe walkers. When they learn to run, they may waddle or not keep up with their peers. When they get up from the ground, they may walk their hands up their legs in what is referred to as a Gower's maneuver. In DMD and BMD, the calves may be large out of proportion to other muscles.

For those with teenage or adult onset, athletics become difficult. Running, getting up from a chair, and going up stairs may become problematic. The individual may notice that muscles are becoming smaller or atrophic. In FSHD, initial signs may be the lack of a smile or "winging" of the scapula when the arms are extended. In DM, the inability to release the grip, called myotonia, may be the first sign. Tripping and falls may be an early sign.

Finally, the initial sign for some patients may be an abnormal blood test. Aspartate aminotransferase (AST) and alanine aminotransferase (ALT) are enzymes commonly assessed in blood tests called **liver function tests**. Levels of these enzymes are abnormal when liver is damaged or inflamed. However, AST and ALT are also made in muscle and are elevated in many MDs in the absence of any liver abnormality. Occasionally, an MD patient will be sent to a gastroenterologist or even have a liver biopsy because of abnormalities in AST and ALT.

A more specific test for muscle is **creatine kinase (CK)**. CK is an intracellular enzyme that is released to the

Developmental delay

A condition in which a child is not developing or achieving skills according to the expected time frame.

Liver function tests

A set of laboratory tests that is used to determine the health of the liver, but are also frequently abnormal in MD.

Creatine kinase (CK)

An intracellular enzyme that is elevated in the blood in some forms of MD.

bloodstream with muscle cell damage. It is massively elevated in some MDs (e.g., DMD, BMD, some LGMD) and is slightly elevated or even normal in others (FSHD, DM).

If you or your child is experiencing weakness or developmental delay, talk to your internist or pediatrician about your concerns. Ask him/her to draw a CK and possibly refer you to a neurologist.

Vicky's Comment:

We first noticed signs at the age of 5, when our son had a unique way of walking and running that differed from other kids his age and then later when he started tiptoe walking. We were told by doctors that he had tight muscles and that intense PT and bilateral casting would help. When none of these showed improvement, and he was tiring faster, we had a blood test done to check his CK level. The results were alarmingly high and that is when our Duchenne journey began.

Lilleen's Comment:

Since I personally had FSHD myself, I knew what signs to look for in my son. It was when he was about 18 months when we took him in for a photo op, that I noticed he had less of a smile. I continued to watch his smile disappear over several months. By the time he was 3, he had completely lost all his facial expressions. I also noticed that when he would walk, he walked on the balls of his feet. Looking back, there were earlier signs, but as a mother, I think I was in denial. When my son was born, his eyes didn't close all the way, and feeding him seemed to take an awful long time. He took forever to finish a bottle, which now I know was due to his poor ability to suck.

Colin's Comment:

Prior to my diagnosis of MD, there were several initial signs that I didn't recognize for what they were. Looking back, I think one of the first signs was severe fatigue, which was exacerbated by my sleep apnea. Other signs such as male pattern baldness and a weakening hand grip I didn't think were symptoms of anything. Another early sign was developing cataracts in both eyes in my early twenties. It wasn't until my father was diagnosed with DM that I found out that all these things were symptoms of DM.

3. How is muscular dystrophy diagnosed?

Generally, people with MD first come to a **neurologist** with muscle weakness. A neurologist is a doctor who has had specialty training in the nervous system including muscle. Some neurologists further specialize in the care of MD patients. Although pain may be a symptom of the individual, pain is usually not the predominant feature.

The neurologist will do a physical exam that includes an assessment of muscle tone and strength, sensation, and reflexes. From this exam, he or she can usually determine if the weakness is coming from muscle or from the nerves, spinal cord, or brain. The neurologist may be aided by some laboratory tests, including a CK level. This is a muscle enzyme released into the bloodstream during muscle damage and is frequently elevated in MD. Sometimes the neurologist will perform **electromyography (EMG),** which consists of electrical recording from various muscles with a fine needle.

Once the diagnosis of a muscle disorder has been made then the neurologist must decide whether the disorder is hereditary or acquired (caused by something other than genetics). MDs are hereditary or genetic disorders. He or she will ask whether anyone else in the extended family has similar symptoms. However, there is often no family history in cases of MD. In such cases, the pattern of muscle involvement and the age of onset and speed of progression can serve as clues whether the symptoms are coming from an acquired disorder (such as inflammation of the muscle or myositis) or a hereditary disorder (such as MD).

Finally, the neurologist must determine which of the dozens of MDs is responsible. The clinical clues described above direct the neurologist in genetic testing. For this testing, a small sample of blood or saliva is used to examine many different genes related to MD. Frequently that leads to a specific diagnosis. On some occasions, the first genetic test does not find the diagnosis. In this situation, he or she may order exome sequencing (ES), which is a test that sequences all the genes in the human genome to look for mutations (see Question 10). Muscle biopsy, although common in the past, is rarely used these days when a neurologist suspects MD, because genetic testing is very good at finding the diagnosis.

With the genetic diagnosis, the neurologist is able to make some general prognoses and plan of care. The diagnosis can be devastating or reassuring. In situations where the **prognosis** is one of a severely disabling and fatal disorder, the news will forever change the dreams and expectations of a family. How that news is delivered, conveying the hope that current research brings, is instrumental in how a family copes with the diagnosis.

Prognosis

A prediction of how the disease will progress.

On the other hand, sometimes the diagnosis puts a name to a long-standing series of mysterious symptoms and can be reassuring to the individual with MD and family.

Vicky's Comment:

The day my son was diagnosed is a day I will never forget. My whole world fell apart, and the long and convoluted journey of finding out that my son had a rare and progressive disease that would one day put him in a wheelchair and ultimately take his life had just begun. It has been a challenging road filled with emotions of denial, anger, resentment, resignation, and finally passion and drive to beat this disease—because it's your child, and nothing gets in the way of protecting him at any cost. Partner that with the best medical professionals committed to finding a cure and an active and supportive Duchenne community that has changed the landscape of the disease, and suddenly there's hope for a future that gives our kids a longer, healthier, and more productive life.

Lilleen's Comment:

Finding out that I had FSHD, although scary, meant that I knew what I was dealing with was not psychological. I had been misdiagnosed with depression for 8 years. Now I knew what was causing my pain and weakness. I felt more in control over how I would deal with my future. Staying positive is one of the ways I choose to combat my disease.

Colin's Comment:

I'll never forget the way I felt when I was diagnosed with DM. I felt lost, hopeless, and very, very angry. It took me years to come to terms with living with DM. It was a struggle, but eventually I was able to accept my situation, and I found the determination to make the best of it. This included rediscovering my passion for sailing and the introduction to a whole community of adaptive sailors—who are sailors first, and disabled second. Not letting my disease define me was a new goal that I strove for. Yes, DM is something I have, but it is not the most interesting thing about me.

4. How do I find good medical care?

Finding a good medical team that specializes in the care of MD is one of the most important things that you can do to care for yourself or your child. It may require some shopping around. Although it is tempting to see the most convenient provider, finding the right team may require travel to another city or state. This can be costly in terms of time and finances, but it may be worth the investment.

I stress the word "team" because that is what is required to provide expert care for the individual with MD. Ideally, the team works together to provide interdisciplinary care on the same day in the same location. This is not always feasible, however, and sometimes it is necessary to construct one's own team from various providers and locations that at a minimum communicate well with each other to develop a consistent plan of treatment.

The first thing to evaluate in your team is the clinic coordinator. Is this person responsive to your needs? Does he or she provide you with information about the medical facility and area and provide you with a written schedule of the providers that you or your child will be seeing? You will have a lot of interactions with this coordinator, and it is essential that he or she is friendly and approachable.

Next, you need to evaluate the central healthcare provider. This is usually a neurologist but can be a physiatrist, geneticist, cardiologist, or pulmonologist. The central healthcare provider needs to be fluent in MD, and if a neurologist or **physiatrist** (a specialist in physical rehabilitation), must have specialty training in neuromuscular disorders. It is worth asking how many years the physician has been in practice and how many patients with your specific MD he or she sees in any given year. It is necessary that the central healthcare provider is willing to learn, is accessible, and truly cares for you or your child. The central healthcare provider should work with a physical therapist (PT) and occupational therapist (OT) who will evaluate you on the same day to provide information on exercises, stretching, bracing, recommendations for **activities of daily living (ADLs)**, and equipment. Ideally, the clinic will also offer a genetics counselor to answer questions of reproduction, inheritance, and genetic testing and a social worker to screen for life stressors and provide guidance on insurance, employment, and schools. Finally, depending on your MD and associated symptoms, the ideal clinic will also have a cardiologist to monitor heart function, initiate preventative measures, and manage cardiomyopathy and arrhythmias and a pulmonologist to monitor lung function, prescribe preventative measures, and manage ventilatory support. The clinic should be able to refer you to an endocrinologist, gastroenterologist, psychiatrist, and nutritionists with experience in MD as the needs arise.

Another important aspect of your medical team is your primary care provider. This doctor will be responsible

Physiatrist

A specialist in physical rehabilitation.

Activities of daily living (ADLs)

Activities that everyone participates in day to day, such as dressing, eating, personal hygiene, grooming, and so forth.

for making sure you or your child's immunizations are up to date and will monitor and manage other health issues. Your neurologist and primary care provider should communicate often.

Luckily, there are several MD clinics across the country that provide expert interdisciplinary care. Many of these are funded by the Muscular Dystrophy Association (MDA) and can be located on their website (https://www.mda.org/care/mda-care-centers). For DMD, Parent Project Muscular Dystrophy (PPMS) evaluates and endorses interdisciplinary clinics, which follow published standards of care guidelines as Certified Duchenne Care Centers (https://www.parentprojectmd.org/care/find-a-certified-duchenne-care-center/). For FSHD, DM, and LGMD, a call to the respective foundations (see Appendix B) may be helpful to locate a center of excellence.

Finally, talk to other families about their experiences. Deciding on the right clinic for you or your child is an important decision that requires some investigation.

Tayjus' Comment:

When it came to finding the right care team, my parents were usually guided by other families and patient advocacy groups like PPMD. I usually would have a clinic close to where I lived in case I needed immediate care, and then another for more advanced care. In a sense, it was a great way to get two opinions. One challenge has been finding a good primary care doctor. While patients with DMD likely have a strong care team for their diagnosis, it is still important to have a primary care doctor. Of course, finding the right care can be a challenge for individuals in more remote areas or who might be on Medicaid or have financial limitations. I think patient advocacy groups are the best to guide patients by designating various clinics as centers of excellence.

Vicky's Comment:

We went to two other clinics before we finally decided on our current clinic. The team here is friendly, compassionate, and professional. The staff is thorough, and each appointment is carefully scheduled so that we are able to meet all our specialists in one day and then have an overview with our primary neurologist. After each specialist appointment, results are discussed and compared to previous visits, then an action plan is devised and evaluated for pros and cons. What I especially like is, now that my son is almost 17 years old, the team really talks to him like an adult, outlining risk–benefit and allowing him to participate in his own care. Finding the right care center has made all the difference in feeling like we are all on one team looking out for my child's best interest.

Lilleen's Comment:

Finding a clinic that not only specialized in FSHD but also one that would see both pediatric and adult patients was of utmost importance to our family, since both my son and I have FSHD. At the time my son was diagnosed, he was only five, and although there were other clinics, I could take him to, they only saw children. The other clinics of choice for myself only saw adults. I needed a place that both my son and I could go to on the same day. I also wanted a place where I knew my son could continue his treatments as an adult. It's hard enough to find good care—no one wants to start over as an adult. My son has seen the same doctor now for over 15 years. So although it may take an hour or more to drive to our clinic, we have always made it a fun time going out to lunch or doing a little sightseeing. Finding a clinic or doctor has to be more than what is convenient. It has to make sense, it has to be about the best care, and it has to be about trusting that you or family are in good hands.

Colin's Comment:

After my father, my sister, and I were diagnosed with MD, we decided to shop around for the best treatment. We went to two or three places but couldn't really find the right fit. Finally, a family friend suggested a clinic—and twenty years later, we're still going there. The team approach is so different from medical care I was familiar with and it has proved to be the best way for dealing with our MD. It is amazing to work with doctors who are not only top in their fields but also experts at how MD affects the different systems of the body. Being part of a family where three out of four are dealing with MD, it was important to find a clinic that could treat us as individuals and as a family. Also, we needed a place where we could all have our appointments at the same time. There is a lot to be said for seeing the same team of doctors every year as your MD progresses and the relationship that developed is equally as important as the medical care we receive.

5. What should I expect at a neurology appointment?

The neurologist is frequently your central healthcare provider. He or she is the one to provide you with your earliest evaluations and diagnosis. He or she will follow you over time, managing your neurological symptoms, coordinating your care with other healthcare providers, and giving you guidance as to what to expect.

It is good to know what to anticipate at your first appointment. The appointment typically begins with a conversation in which the neurologist takes your **history**. This includes an understanding of how the disease started, how it is progressing, and what are the predominant current symptoms. The neurologist will also want to know about your general medical health and past surgical history. He or she will ask you about your family history in order to determine how this may have been inherited. Finally, the neurologist will ask you about school, employment, living situation, sexual orientation, gender identity, and substance use in what is called the social history. This helps the neurologist understand what factors may be impacted by or affecting the disorder.

The appointment then moves to the physical examination. This will begin with a general medical exam in which the physician will evaluate the heart, lungs, and abdomen. Next is the neurological examination. The first time you see the neurologist, he or she will assess your thinking (the mental status exam) and some specialized nerves (the cranial nerve exam). This won't necessarily happen at every visit, as these are rarely affected in MD. The physician will then take a good look at your various muscles. One of the things that he or she is evaluating is whether there is any increased or decreased size of the muscles. The neurologist will then evaluate the strength of various muscles in the neck, limbs, and trunk. This is done by what is called manual muscle testing in which muscles are rated on a scale of 0 (no movement) to 5 (full strength). Some neurologists also evaluate strength by means of **handheld dynamometry** in which you push against an instrument that measures the force of your muscles. It is

History

An assessment of individual's current health as well as information of past medical conditions, family health, and social factors that may impact health.

Handheld dynamometry

A test of muscle strength used to measure the force of muscles.

very helpful for the neurologist to also have timed function tests, such as the time for your child to get up off the floor, the time for you to run 10 meters, or the time for you to climb four stairs. Sometimes, the neurologist will have these timed function tests done by the physical therapist who works with him or her (see **Figure 1**). The neurologist will watch you walk or run. He or she will assess your sensation (also not affected in MD) and finally your reflexes. From this examination, the neurologist is able to determine the pattern of weakness and over time, the rate of progression.

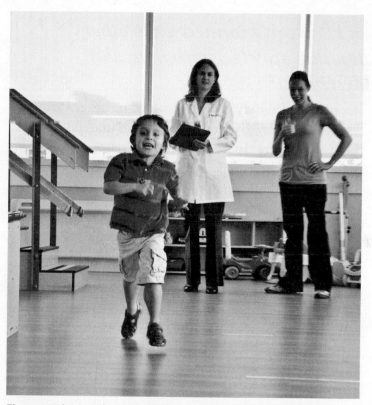

Figure 1 A young boy with DMD performing a timed function test: The 10-meter run.

After the initial examination, the neurologist will provide you with an assessment including a likely diagnosis. He or she will recommend next steps, including diagnostic testing. At subsequent visits, there will be recommendations for treatment, physical therapy, nutrition, bracing, and equipment, to name some examples. It is generally recommended that boys with DMD see their neurologist every 6 months and those with adult-onset MD see their neurologist once a year. For those who have very slowly progressive MD, a visit every 2 years for monitoring and anticipatory guidance may be sufficient.

6. How can I connect with other families affected with muscular dystrophy?

It can be extremely helpful to talk to others affected by MD for peer-to-peer support. You understand that there are others in very similar circumstances. You share stories. You pick up tips for care. You compare notes. Although it may not be obvious where to find others with a rare disease, there are several avenues.

Register with a patient foundation. Some of these are listed in Appendix B. Many of these foundations organize support groups (e.g., MDA and Myotonic), educational events (e.g., FSHD Society), or online communities (e.g., PPMD). Some organize conferences devoted to care considerations and research (e.g., PPMD and CureDuchenne) where you can meet other families with the disease and learn about recent advancements.

Consider participating in a fundraising event. These events not only raise funds for much needed research in MD but bring together people for a fun activity.

Connect online. There are many existing Facebook groups, or you could start your own.

Make peer connections. Talk to your neurologist or clinic social worker about others living with the disease in your area. Your healthcare provider will need the permission of both families to connect you for privacy reasons. This can be a wonderful way to meet someone with the same disease in the same geographic area. And if your child has MD, send him or her to MDA camp or Camp Promise! These one-week camps allow your child to meet others with neuromuscular disease while gaining some independence and having fun in a variety of specially structured activities.

Tayjus' Comment:

Having other friends with MD has always been a huge resource. You have a community to ask questions about what doctor to see, or how to travel, or how to find personal care assistants. For my family, I think we were able to connect with a local family through a patient advocacy group, and this family was so helpful in guiding my parents in regard to all the benefits out there for families like ours. Of course, today with the internet it is so easy to find other families with MD, to the point where it can be overwhelming. There are so many Facebook groups out there for a newly diagnosed family to join, for families with children in clinical trials, or even for patients transitioning into adulthood. I also know of many families who have made lifelong friends from meeting other families at the neuromuscular clinic during their doctor's appointment. Today, I can honestly say that I am part of a DMD family. I may not see them every day, but it is so great to see the amazing things people are doing in spite of MD.

Vicky's Comment:

Finding other families that share this journey had been very helpful for us. Organizations such as MDA and PPMD have been excellent resources for connecting us to other families and for providing information. They sponsor different events that connect people in any way associated with DMD.

Lilleen's Comment:

I was an adult at the time I attended my first FSHD meeting. I had never met anyone else with FSHD, so I didn't know where to turn to or who to talk to about what I was experiencing. I soon found a group of very supportive people where I learned so much from others who had experienced similar situations. At first it was hard to see how each person was affected, some not as advanced and others very advanced. I had no idea how different this disease could affect each individual. It can be very difficult to see someone else in a wheelchair for the first time, and wonder is that one's future. A few years later, I went from attending a group to hosting my own social gathering with the FSHD Society. So if you can't find a support group in your area, don't be afraid of creating your own.

PART TWO

Genetics

How did I get this disease?

Should I have genetic testing?

What kinds of genetic testing are available?

More . . .

7. How did I get this disease?

MDs are genetic conditions, meaning that they are caused by changes or errors in a person's genes. Genes are the instructions for our bodies to grow, develop, and function. Genes are made up of DNA, which is like a series of letters that spell out the instructions. DNA and genes are packaged into structures called chromosomes that are located in the nucleus or core of each cell and passed down from parent to child. We have 23 pairs of chromosomes, 46 total, that are numbered 1 to 22—the last pair is the sex chromosomes, X and Y. Females have two X chromosomes, and males have an X and a Y. We inherit one copy of each chromosome pair (and therefore one copy of each gene) from our mother and one copy from our father. Changes in the genetic instructions—such as DNA misspellings, extra or missing chromosome material, or alterations in how genes are expressed—can result in problems with development and/or functioning in the individual, depending on which gene or genes are affected. Many, but not all, of the genes involved in MD code for a protein that gives structure to the muscle cell. An error in one of these genes causes a loss of function of the muscle protein.

There are several different inheritance patterns for MDs.

Autosomal dominant MDs are caused by genes on the numbered chromosomes (every person has two copies of the gene), and the disease occurs if *one* copy of the gene is erroneous. Examples of autosomal dominant MDs include FSHD, OPMD, DM, some LGMD, and some DD. In these disorders it is common to see MD in grandparents, parents, and children.

Autosomal recessive MDs are also caused by genes on the numbered chromosomes, but unlike autosomal dominant MD the disease only occurs if *both* gene copies are erroneous. Parents of a person with an autosomal recessive MD are usually carriers of one abnormal gene, but they do not manifest MD because the other copy of the gene is normal. In these families, you do not see multiple generations affected although you may see siblings affected. This can explain why an individual has MD with no family history of the disease.

X-linked MDs are caused by genes on the X chromosome and usually only affect males, since males only have one X chromosome. Females can be carriers of an X-linked MD but usually do not show symptoms, since females have a second gene copy that is normal. Occasionally, females can show milder symptoms of MD, which is called being a **manifesting carrier**. Males with X-linked MD often inherit the condition from their mother (since males get their one X chromosome from their mother). Males pass on their X chromosome to their daughters who would be carriers and at risk of having affected sons of their own (grandsons of an affected male). In families with X-linked MD, we often see affected males related through females.

Manifesting carrier

A female with only one gene for an X-linked type of MD who nevertheless has symptoms of MD.

Genetic changes causing MD may be inherited or occur new ("de novo") in the affected individual. In **de novo cases**, the error is not inherited from the mother or father but appears for the first time in the child. De novo genetic changes happen due to random errors in the cell, usually in the egg or the sperm. There is nothing that a mother or father does to cause de novo changes to happen, and also no known environmental causes. In DMD and FSHD, approximately one-third of all cases are due to de novo mutations. This is another reason why an individual can have MD without any family history of the disease.

De novo case

The occurrence of a genetic disease for the first time in a family with no history of the disease.

The inheritance of DM1 is unique. As a bit of background, genes are composed of four specific chemical components called nucleotides, which are named adenine, cytosine, guanine, and thymine. In describing a gene, those nucleotides are represented by the letters A, C, G, and T, which are used to "spell out" the gene's sequence. DM1 is an autosomal dominant disorder in which a part of the affected gene has DNA nucleotides that are repeated multiple times. Having too many of these "repeats" causes the gene to work differently. The number of repeats sometimes increases when passed from parent to child, such that each successive generation has larger and larger expansions. Larger expansions are associated with earlier and more severe disease. Therefore, the grandparent may have very mild disease, the parent may have moderate disease, and the child may have severe **congenital disease**. Sometimes a child is diagnosed before a parent because of this difference across generations. OPMD is also an autosomal dominant disorder due to a repeat expansion. However, OPMD does not have expanding repeat size with successive generations.

Congenital disease
Disease present at birth.

It is important that you understand the inheritance of your specific form of MD so that you can make important family planning decisions and so that you can identify those at risk for inheriting the disorder. Your genetic counselor can provide you with this information (Question 14).

8. Should I have genetic testing?

If you or a family member is affected with MD, one of the questions that you will need to think carefully about is whether you want to have genetic testing. There are several benefits to testing, but also some potential risks. Your genetics counselor will discuss these with you.

Genetic testing has the potential to provide you with information about whether you have a specific MD, are at risk of developing an MD, or are a carrier of MD. There are several advantages to having a specific diagnosis. The information that a specific diagnosis provides may guide management of your disorder. If there are specific treatments for your condition, it will provide rationale for starting such a treatment. It may also help protect you from being put on a treatment for another condition that would not be helpful. It is important to know if you have a type of MD that can affect other body systems, such as cardiac or pulmonary, so that you can be monitored for those potential complications. Carriers of DMD, for instance, are at increased risk for **cardiomyopathy** and should begin cardiac screening in late adolescence or early adulthood—or earlier, if they have signs or symptoms of a heart disorder. Undergoing genetic testing may allow your healthcare professionals to tailor your treatment and management to your disorder.

Cardiomyo-pathy

A disorder of the heart muscle.

For many of the MDs, there is no specific treatment. The information provided by a specific diagnosis can still be helpful in terms of providing you with a prognosis. Your healthcare professionals can compare your progression to that of others they have been treating with the disorder and help you better anticipate the future.

A specific genetic diagnosis is required for most clinical trials in MD. You may or may not wish to participate in a clinical study or trial (see Question 29), but having a specific diagnosis gives you the option to participate. If you have a specific diagnosis, then you can participate in one of several disease-specific registries. These registries will often notify you of upcoming studies and trials that you are eligible for.

Having a specific diagnosis allows you to understand the inheritance of your disease (see Question 7) and your risk of passing it on (see Question 11). This is important information for making decisions about family planning. It is also incredibly helpful information for your extended family to understand their risks.

There are also some potential risks to genetic testing. One type of risk is the emotional impact of results. Research has shown that most people do not experience long-lasting negative reactions to receiving genetic test results; however, some individuals do find the information emotionally troubling. For example, a mother of a boy with DMD may wish to know if she is a carrier for family planning purposes and for understanding her own health risks. However, she may experience feelings of guilt to learn that she passed on a gene that causes disease in her son. As another example, a young person with minimal symptoms may be troubled to learn definitively that he or she has a progressive MD.

On the other hand, some people may have positive emotional reactions. For example, a person who has been experiencing unexplained symptoms may feel relief to finally have a diagnosis. Likewise, a person with a family history of MD likely will be relieved to receive a negative result that means they are not at risk or a carrier. Often, there is a mix of positive and negative emotions. It is important that you consider how you may feel about results, assess your current mental health, and have good support networks before launching into genetic testing. A genetic counselor (Question 14) can provide short-term emotional support and help with decision making about genetic testing. If you need longer term support, you may wish to see a therapist.

Several laws protect individuals who have had genetic testing. This includes the Genetic Information Nondiscrimination Act (GINA) of 2008 that states that an employer cannot use genetic information for hiring, firing, or promotions and that health insurance companies cannot use it as an exclusionary preexisting condition. Important limitations of GINA are that it does not apply to employers with fewer than 15 employees or individuals covered by some forms of federal and military insurance. In addition, GINA does not apply to life, long-term care, or disability insurance. You may wish to secure this insurance before you have genetic testing. The Affordable Care Act of 2010 prohibits issuers of health insurance from discriminating against patients with genetic conditions. There are other federal and state laws that offer protections. More information about laws related to genetic discrimination can be found here: https://www.genome.gov/about-genomics/policy-issues/Genetic-Discrimination.

9. What kinds of genetic testing are available?

There are many different kinds of genetic testing. Which one is most appropriate for you depends on what diseases are being considered and what information is already available on a family's health history. If there is a strong clinical suspicion of a specific MD, then a **single gene test** may be ordered. This blood test will give information only on whether the individual is

Single gene test

A genetic test that assesses an individual gene associated with the specific type of MD for which there is strong clinical suspicion.

at risk of developing this one disease. If an individual has symptoms that are common to several MDs such as the LGMDs or DD, then a **gene panel** may be recommended. Panels typically include many genes (ranging from less than 5 to several dozen or more) associated with groups of MDs and can provide information on several MDs. An alternative to panel testing is exome sequencing (ES) (discussed further in Question 10) that provides information on even a larger number of genes.

Gene panel

A genetic testing strategy that reviews multiple genes that are associated with MD.

If one family member has tested positive for a specific MD, then other family members can have targeted variant testing. This testing utilizes the specific information that is available for the affected individual and only tests to determine if the same variant is found in family members. This testing will not reveal whether the family member has another genetic error, although the risk of another genetic error causing MD is low.

The cost of genetic testing has decreased significantly in recent years. Most insurance companies now cover genetic testing, although there may be requirements such as preauthorization and/or having the test done at a particular laboratory. Before you have a genetic test, your doctor or genetic counselor should help you determine insurance coverage. The costs of genetic testing vary depending on which test is ordered. Targeted variant and single-gene genetic tests are typically less expensive than panel or ES.

Your doctor or genetic counselor (Question 14) will guide you in the most appropriate test for your situation. It is best to have a genetic counselor involved for complicated scenarios and ES.

10. What is exome sequencing?

Exome sequencing (ES), also known as Whole Exome Sequencing (WES), is a relatively new tool that has been incredibly helpful in providing a diagnosis to patients with MD. Sometimes, the physician who evaluates you or your child will have a good sense of which gene is affected based on the clinical presentation and can order testing specific for that MD. Other times, it will be less clear, and a wider net needs to be cast. This is when ES comes into play.

Our chromosomes are composed of DNA, some of which encodes for proteins that give us our unique characteristics. Not all DNA encodes for proteins, however. Only about 1–2% of all DNA encodes for proteins. These protein-coding regions of genes are called **exons**. The **exome** refers to the entire collection of exons in an individual's **genome**. ES is a technique in which the exons of nearly all of a person's genes can be rapidly sequenced by a process called next generation sequencing from a few tablespoons of blood or even a cheek swab or saliva sample. While the exome only makes up a small percentage of our total DNA, the majority (about 85%) of genetic changes that cause inherited diseases are located in the exome. ES is therefore an efficient way to search for the genetic cause of a person's condition.

Exons
The protein-coding regions of genes.

Exome
The full collection of exons in an individual's genome.

Genome
All of the genetic material of an individual.

ES is a powerful tool that can provide a wealth of data. It is able to evaluate many genes at once and thus help identify an MD from many possibilities. Currently, ES is able to identify the specific diagnosis in about 25% of people with MD. When possible, an individual's parents are included in ES, because this increases the likelihood of finding the diagnosis and decreases the chance of generating uncertain results.

As with any genetic test, there are limitations of ES. Some types of genetic changes cannot be detected by ES. Importantly ES cannot detect disorders such as DM and OPMD that are caused by DNA repeats, nor can ES detect the complex genetic changes associated with FSHD. Another limitation to ES is that it does not look at DNA in noncoding regions, so if your MD is caused by a genetic change outside of the exome, it would not be found on ES. Also, we believe there are genetic types of MD that have not yet been discovered, so a person may have a negative ES result because their specific form of MD is caused by a gene that is not yet known. It is therefore important that you continue to follow-up with your doctor or genetic counselor in the future, even if you have a negative ES result. Many genetic testing laboratories offer ES "reanalysis," which would take into account new gene discoveries. Also, more advanced testing such as genome sequencing may become routinely clinically available in the future.

Another challenge with ES is determining the meaning or significance of genetic changes. Every person has tens of thousands of differences (variants) in his or her DNA, most of which do not cause any problem. Sometimes it is obvious when a particular DNA change is the cause of a person's condition; this is called a *pathogenic variant* or a mutation. Other times, a variant may be found in a gene associated with MD, but it is not known whether that particular variant is causative or whether it could simply be a benign or normal variation. This type of result is called a **variant of unknown significance** or **VUS**. It can be frustrating to have a VUS because there may be a suggestion that you have a specific type of MD, but it cannot be

Variant of unknown significance (VUS)

A genetic variation in a gene that cannot be definitively determined as causing or not causing MD.

determined conclusively at that time. Thanks to new research, knowledge about the meaning of genetic variants is increasing, so in the future your doctor or genetic counselor may be able to determine the meaning of your VUS. It is very important to periodically follow up with a genetic counselor about your results.

Because ES is testing nearly all of your genes, not just MD genes, there is the potential to learn information that is not related to your MD but might be important for your health; this is called *secondary findings* or *incidental findings*. If you have ES, you usually will be given the choice to learn if you have certain other genetic conditions that are potentially preventable or treatable if caught early. These conditions include hereditary cancer syndromes (such as the *BRCA* genes associated with high risk for breast and other cancers) and certain inherited heart conditions such as cardiomyopathy. ES on rare occasions has revealed unexpected information about family relationships—for example, an adopted child who was never told that he was adopted might discover that he was unrelated to his parents, or a father might discover that his son or daughter is not his biological offspring.

In summary, ES is a powerful new test method that can provide genetic diagnoses for many people with MD. This has benefits for the patient and their family members who may be carriers or at risk of the disease. It also has limitations such as unclear results as in the example of VUS. And finally, there are risks such as additional upsetting information. If ES is recommended to you, it is important that you meet with a genetic counselor both before and after your testing to understand these benefits, limitations, and risks and to fully understand the implications of your results (see Question 14).

11. Can I pass muscular dystrophy on to my children?

Many individuals with MD or carriers of MD are concerned about passing the disease onto their children. To understand this risk, it is important to have a specific genetic diagnosis (see Question 8) and to understand the inheritance pattern for that specific diagnosis (see **Figure 2A-C** below).

For individuals with an autosomal dominant MD (DM, FSHD, OPMD, some LGMD, some DD) the risk of passing on the abnormal gene to their child is 50-50, like flipping a coin. This means that in each pregnancy conceived by a person with an autosomal dominant MD, there is a 50% chance that the child will inherit the abnormal gene and be affected by (or at risk of) the MD, and a 50% chance that the child will inherit the normal gene and be unaffected. Importantly, the probability of passing on the abnormal gene is independent in each pregnancy. If there are two children, they may both be affected, both be unaffected, or one affected and the other unaffected. Children who inherit the abnormal gene are at risk of developing the disease. It is important to remember, however, that children may not have the same severity of disease as their parents. For DM1, the severity increases, and the age of onset decreases with each generation. For FSHD, there is wide variability in the severity among affected individuals in the same family, and some people who inherited the abnormal gene may never show any symptoms (nonmanifesting carriers).

For individuals affected with autosomal recessive MD (most CMD, many LGMD, some DD), all of their children will be carriers of one abnormal gene copy, but the only way they could be affected is if they inherit an abnormal gene copy from both parents. Most types of MD are rare, so the likelihood that the other parent could be a carrier is low. The other parent could choose to have genetic testing to determine if they are a carrier. If one parent has an autosomal recessive MD and the other parent is a carrier, there is a 50% risk for each child to be affected with MD. For parents of an individual affected with an autosomal recessive MD, both parents are usually carriers, and there is a 25% chance in each pregnancy that the child will inherit an abnormal gene from both parents and be affected with MD.

For female carriers of an X-linked disorder (mothers or sisters of DMD, some EDMD), the risk of passing the abnormal gene onto their child is similarly 50-50. If the child is a girl and inherits the abnormal gene, she will be a carrier. Carriers can be unaffected or have milder symptoms of the disorder. If the child who inherits the abnormal gene is a boy, he will be affected with MD.

For men with an X-linked disorder (DMD, some EDMD), none of their sons will be affected, since sons inherit the father's Y chromosome and a normal gene copy from their mother. Daughters of men with X-linked MD will always be carriers, since they inherit their father's X chromosome with the abnormal gene.

As you can see, the answer to this question depends heavily on the type of MD that you have and its mode of inheritance. Your genetic counselor can help you understand these risks (Question 14).

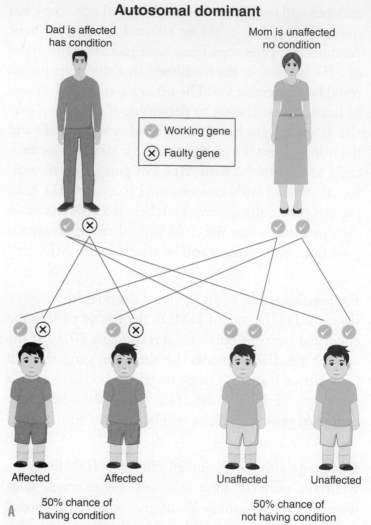

Autosomal dominant

Dad is affected
has condition

Mom is unaffected
no condition

✓ Working gene
✗ Faulty gene

Affected

Affected

Unaffected

Unaffected

A   50% chance of
having condition

50% chance of
not having condition

Figure 2 (A) Autosomal dominant, **(B)** autosomal recessive.
(C) X-linked recessive (*Continued*)

Illustrations courtesy of Arjun Ramesh.

Autosomal recessive

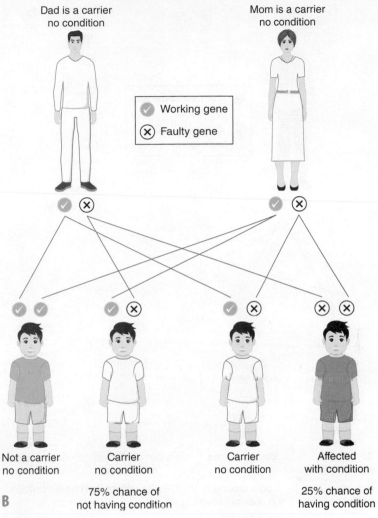

Dad is a carrier
no condition

Mom is a carrier
no condition

✓ Working gene
✗ Faulty gene

Not a carrier
no condition

Carrier
no condition

Carrier
no condition

Affected
with condition

75% chance of
not having condition

25% chance of
having condition

B

Figure 2 *(Continued)*

Illustrations courtesy of Arjun Ramesh.

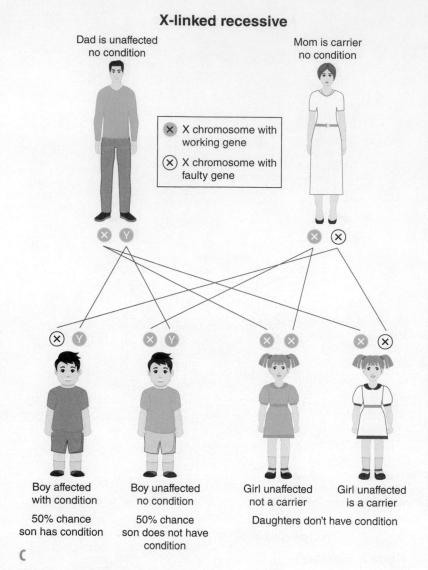

X-linked recessive

Dad is unaffected
no condition

Mom is carrier
no condition

⊗ X chromosome with
working gene

⊗ X chromosome with
faulty gene

Boy affected
with condition

Boy unaffected
no condition

Girl unaffected
not a carrier

Girl unaffected
is a carrier

50% chance
son has condition

50% chance
son does not have
condition

Daughters don't have condition

C

Figure 2 (Continued)

Illustrations courtesy of Arjun Ramesh.

12. Should my child have genetic testing?

The decision to test a child is somewhat different from the decision to test oneself or an adult (see Question 8). There are several questions to ask when deciding to test a child:

- *Does the child exhibit symptoms of disease?* For a child with developmental delay or weakness, it is usually helpful to have a genetic diagnosis. This can end the diagnostic odyssey in which the family goes from one healthcare provider to another in search of an understanding of the symptoms. The genetic diagnosis may also lead to specific disease treatments and monitoring, as is the case in DMD where there are published guidelines for the standard of care. However, if the child does not exhibit symptoms of disease but rather is at risk for inheriting the disease with a later onset, it may be prudent to avoid early testing. Current ethical guidelines agree that in most cases, genetic testing should not be performed on asymptomatic minors when there are no effective measures to prevent, treat, or ameliorate the disease, as is the case for many MDs. An early diagnosis may adversely affect parenting or self-fulfillment and takes away the autonomy of making the decision to be tested as an adult. Deferring testing until adulthood allows children to make their own informed decisions.

- *Is the child sexually active?* For a child at risk of inheriting MD and passing on the gene, it may be helpful for family planning purposes to have genetic testing. This is an area that many parents and adolescents are uncomfortable exploring together. Adolescents should have the opportunity for confidential discussions with doctors and genetic counselors without the presence of their parents.

- *Is the child in good mental health?* The results of genetic testing can have a significant psychological impact. If the test is positive for an MD, this can change the way the child perceives his or her future and abilities. If the test is negative, there may be guilt associated with being free of the disease while other family members are affected. Testing is usually not an urgent issue and should be done when the child is well supported and is relatively free of anxiety and depression.

- *Does the child agree to testing?* Depending on the age of the child, it is important to get his or her buy-in to genetic testing in an age-appropriate fashion. This is information that will travel with the child for a lifetime and influence decisions that he or she makes.

Genetic counselors (Question 14) can help parents work through the decision to test their child, assist in explaining the testing in an age-appropriate fashion, and provide support through the process.

13. How do I tell my child that he or she has muscular dystrophy?

Most parents wish to protect their child from distress and, in attempting to do so, may be reluctant to talk to their child about their diagnosis. However, it is important that you do so in an age-appropriate fashion. Your child already knows that there is something wrong with his or her body and has noticed symptoms, such as not keeping up with peers, frequent medical appointments, and family stress and distress related to the child's health. Without accurate information, children may think that their parents are upset because of something they did wrong or may have feelings of inadequacy (despite your reassurances to the contrary). Your child may feel that the problem is too horrible to talk about, and that by not talking, he or she can protect *you* from distress. Children often pick up on deception, and deception communicates to them that we don't trust them or think they are not capable of handling the truth. Talking about MD helps correct any wrong assumptions, takes away feelings of guilt, and allows children to ask questions and share their feelings about the problem. It builds trust between you and your child, and between your child and healthcare providers. Everyone is better able to cope with difficult situations when they have information, and children are no different. Even more important, talking about MD gives children the knowledge and vocabulary that they will need in the future to make decisions about their care, advocate for themselves, and inform others. It is the first step in helping them be independent. Remember, our job as parents is not to protect our child from all of life's difficulties, but to teach them how to cope and succeed despite them.

Some parents may wish to delay talking about MD until their child is older, because they believe that the child will be better able to understand or cope with their condition. However, it's better to start talking about MD earlier rather than later, as this "normalizes" things and makes talking about MD less of a big deal. It also allows you to control the flow of information, in that it ensures they are getting good information from the beginning.

How and what you tell your child depends on his or her age and maturity level. For all ages, it is important to let the child's questions guide the discussion. One conversation will not be enough, and your initial conversation is simply setting the stage for future conversations. Don't be afraid of "saying the wrong thing." Although it does not happen as often as you might think, conversations about MD sometimes cause a child to become emotional and upset. This is a normal reaction to a difficult and stressful situation. Do not be too quick to provide false reassurances or minimize their distress. Validating and discussing their feelings help them learn how to cope and adjust. Encourage your child to talk to you and his or her healthcare providers about MD whenever questions arise. Be honest with your child, in a hopeful and positive manner, and don't avoid answering difficult questions.

In the 3–7 age range, it is important to let the child know that the child's muscle weakness is not something that he or she caused but is due to a problem with the muscles called MD that your child was born with. Use clear and simple language. You can reassure your child that the doctors and physical therapists are working to help him/her with this problem and that there are things he or she can do, like stretching and taking medications, that will help this problem. It is helpful for you to not only answer your child's questions but to ask the child to explain back to you what you have said so that you can gauge your child's understanding and clear up any misperceptions or simplify things. Some children may initially deny that they have a problem with their muscles, but that is normal and okay.

Let your child know that not all information on the internet is accurate or up to date.

In the 7–12 age range, you can explain that the weakness your child is experiencing is caused by a problem with muscles called MD, and this problem is caused by a faulty gene that your child was born with. If other family members have this disorder, it may be helpful to reveal this information (if they are positive role models). Your child will be getting information from other sources such as the internet, and it is important that he or she comes to you with questions that arise from this information. You should explain that all MDs are not the same and that not all information is applicable. Also, let your child know that not all information on the internet is accurate or up to date. Reassure your child that there are things that he or she can do to help, such as eating healthy foods, taking medications, and stretching. Let your child know that it is okay to be angry or sad about this problem.

Your teenager will be able to understand more about MD and its inheritance and will have more detailed questions for you. It may be helpful to have an early conversation with your doctor or genetic counselor and your teenager so that all his or her questions are answered (see Question 14). Expect that your teenager will get a lot of information from the internet and make sure the lines of communication are open so that he or she comes to you with questions or disturbing information. Again, explain that all MDs are not the same, and that not all information is relevant or accurate. Include your teenager in decision-making about his or her care so that he or she feels empowered. Emphasize the things that he or she can do to help such as eating healthy foods, taking medications, and stretching, and highlight the teenager's abilities, such as academic pursuits, that are not affected by MD.

For all children, it is important to communicate a sense of hope when discussing a diagnosis. There is so much advancement in research and care of those with MD that future generations will have very different lives than past generations.

Vicky's Comment:

We told our son about his diagnosis over a weekend when he was 6. We shared that he had a condition that made his muscles weak, and this condition occurred only in boys. That explained why his sister wasn't affected, but then he wanted to know why his Dad or any other male in the family didn't have it. He asked a lot of questions throughout the weekend and then kind of moved on with life as normal. At that stage, there were few signs of the disease, but it laid the ground for future conversations as he progressed.

Lilleen's Comment:

My son was about 5 when he came to me and asked why he couldn't smile. Up to this point I had not spoken to him about him having MD. I was waiting until I thought he would better understand. However, he was aware that I had something that caused me to become too weak to run and chase him or get down on the floor to play games with him. I explained to him that he and I were both born with the same thing called MD, and it caused our muscles to get weaker over time, and that some of the muscles affected different parts of our body—and the face/smile was one area that was affected. After that day, we have kept a very open dialogue, and although the questions never get easier, he knows he can come to me and ask me questions or tell me how he is feeling.

14. How can I find a genetic counselor?

A **genetic counselor** is an important member of your healthcare team. Genetic counselors are Master's level health professionals with training in clinical genetics and psychological counseling. Genetic counselors are trained in all aspects of genetics and a broad range of

Genetic Counselor

Genetic counselors provide a critical service to individuals and families considering undergoing genetic testing by helping them identify their risks for certain disorders, investigate family health history, interpret information and determine if testing is needed.

genetic indications, though nowadays many genetic counselors specialize in certain areas, including neuromuscular disorders. Look for a genetic counselor with certification by the American Board of Genetic Counseling. This healthcare professional can provide education about inheritance pattern and recurrence risk, counseling about reproductive options, coordinate appropriate genetic testing and interpretation of results, facilitate testing of relatives, and provide guidance and support throughout the diagnostic process.

Many MD dystrophy clinics have a genetic counselor embedded as part of the team who works closely with the neurologist. If not, the clinic may be able to refer you to a genetic counselor who works in the same medical institution or nearby. You can also locate a genetic counselor yourself through the National Society of Genetic Counselors at www.findageneticcounselor.com. There are also "telegenetics" companies that enable you to receive counseling via telephone or video. Finally, many of the genetic testing companies provide genetic counseling services to help in interpretation of results.

PART THREE

Keeping Muscles Strong

Why are my muscles weak?

How weak will I get?

Is it safe to exercise?

More . . .

15. Why are my muscles weak?

The causes of MD are numerous. Many are due to the loss of a link between the inside and the outside of the muscle cell. When this link is broken, the integrity of the muscle cell membrane disintegrates, and there is muscle cell death. If you were to look at your muscle under a microscope (see **Figure 3**) you would see small or atrophic muscle cells, dying muscle cells, but also new regenerating muscle cells. Unfortunately, the regeneration cannot keep up with the degradation. When this happens, muscle cells are replaced by fat and fibrosis (scar tissue). The common end stage of all MDs is muscle composed of fat. This is different from the fat outside your muscles and cannot be controlled by losing weight. Your muscles are weak because the contractile muscle cells are atrophied and replaced by noncontractile fat.

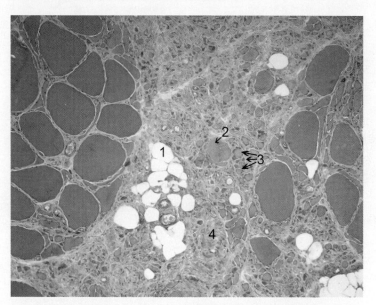

Figure 3 A view from under the microscope of an individual with FSHD. This shows muscle replaced by fat (1), with degenerating fibers (2), many small atrophic fibers (3), and fibrosis or scar tissue (4).

16. How weak will I get?

This outcome is difficult to predict even for your neurologist, who knows you well. The answer may depend on your specific MD, your gene mutation, and your overall health. One way to predict future weakness is to look at the age of symptom onset and the rate of progression. Earlier onset with faster rates of progression will generally lead to more disability than later onset and slower rates of progression.

Progression may mean the involvement of different muscles over time. MDs are characterized by specific patterns of muscle involvement (e.g., FSHD may first affect face, shoulders, and arms); however, over time, the range of muscles affected grows (so that, for example, the leg muscles will also become affected in FSHD). It is not well understood why these patterns of muscle involvement exist and why certain muscles are less affected or spared.

Weakness in MDs does not tend to speed up over time. With notable exceptions—for example, in FSHD, which can have a stepwise progression—the loss of strength is fairly linear from year to year. However, at some point, your weakness progresses so that you cross a functional threshold: you are no longer able to rise from a chair, climb stairs, or walk, for example. This gives the appearance and experience of weakness accelerating.

Many people want to know if they will be able to continue to walk. Walking depends on the strength of multiple muscles in the trunk, hips, and legs as well as balance and overall weight. The quadriceps are particularly important to keep the knee from collapsing. Within the same MD, there are wide variations in the length of time of ambulation. In DMD, children as young as 8 may lose ambulation while others as old as 18 continue walking. However, currently, all boys with DMD will lose the ability to walk. About 20% of all those with FSHD lose the ability to walk. The vast majority of DM patients continue to walk although many with limitations.

These are some generalities, but predicting how weak any specific patient will get is impossible. Meanwhile, there are important steps you can take, including medications, exercise, and nutrition, to keep yourself in your best health and manage your disease. These will be discussed in the following questions and answers.

17. Is it safe to exercise?

It's understandable if you are confused about exercise. The medical community has changed its mind several times about the safety and efficacy of exercise for those with MD. There are still very few clinical trials that have evaluated exercise in MD, and these studies have used different training protocols, making it difficult to compare the studies' findings.

Collective reviews of studies have found that there are no adverse effects of exercise.[1] It is unclear if exercise is beneficial with some studies showing enhanced strength and function while others do not.

Consensus guidelines recommend that patients with FSHD engage in low-intensity aerobic exercise.[2] Similarly, consensus guidelines recommend moderate intensity aerobic and resistance training exercise for DM.[3] Expert opinion in DMD recommends regular sub-maximal aerobic activity and exercise.[4] There are many possible exercise routines that meet these guidelines such as swimming or cycling 30 minutes, 3 or 4 times per week. Your physical therapist can help craft a program specifically for you. If you have a cardiologist, talk to him or her prior to starting an exercise program.

There are a few general guidelines about exercise you should follow to keep yourself safe. Your muscles may not regenerate as well from an injury as healthy muscle. Damage to muscle occurs during eccentric contractions defined as when a muscle is asked to bear a load and lengthen at the same time. It is difficult to exercise without any eccentric contractions, but you can minimize them. A trainer or a physical therapist working with you can help. Exercise should not be painful. If your muscles feel tired or are burning, you should stop. If you develop pigmented urine (**myoglobinuria**) within 24 hours after exercising, you know you have overdone it and need to modify your regimen.

Myoglobinuria

Pigmented urine from breakdown of muscle and release of myoglobin into the bloodstream.

Exercise combats atrophy of muscles from disuse, which can be superimposed on muscles weakened from MD. Exercise can also improve flexibility and range of motion of joints. It improves bone density, which is often reduced in MD. Exercise has cardiopulmonary benefits. Finally, exercise has psychological benefits. With a few precautions, you can safely exercise and reap these benefits.

18. What are the goals of physical therapy?

Physical therapy (PT) plays a vital role in management of MD and achieves several goals. Ideally, you

Physical therapy (PT)

The treatment of disease, injury, or deformity by physical methods such as massage, heat treatment, and exercise rather than by drugs or surgery.

should have a PT evaluation during each interdisciplinary clinic visit (approximately every year for adult onset MD and approximately every 6 months for pediatric MD). The physical therapist in your interdisciplinary clinic will provide you with an individualized treatment plan and communicate with your school or community physical therapist for more frequent direct care. Sometimes the physical therapist in clinic is the same physical therapist that you visit multiple times a week for care.

One of the first goals of PT is an assessment of your current status. This includes an assessment of your range of motion across several joints, strength, function, pain, quality of life, and participation in normal ADLs. For children and in clinic, this assessment frequently includes the North Star Ambulatory Assessment, a 17-item rating scale to measure functional motor abilities. The physical therapist will also measure the time it takes to do certain functions such as standing up from a lying down position, running 10 meters, or climbing four stairs. For adults, the physical therapist may measure the time it takes you to get up from a chair, walk, and sit back down (the timed up and go), run 10 meters, or climb four stairs. The physical therapist may also assess the strength of key muscles with manual tests or using special instruments. These assessments are helpful to the interdisciplinary team to monitor clinical progression, assess the effects of therapies and provide prognostic information.

Contractures

Shortening of muscles and tendons, leading to decreased range of motion.

The physical therapist works with you to prevent and minimize progressive **contractures** (shortening of muscles and tendons leading to decreased range of motion). The physical therapist will demonstrate passive stretches gently moving arms and legs and may teach the individual how to perform active stretches—that is, stretching a muscle by actively contracting the muscle in opposition to the one you're stretching—if the individual is able to perform these independently (Figure 4).

Another major goal of therapy is to maintain function and/or improve strength and function and help adapt to any loss of function. The physical therapist will set up an exercise program that is appropriate, not too strenuous or fatiguing. This may involve cycling or **aquatic therapy,** for instance. In aquatic therapy, the buoyancy of the water assists mobility. In addition, water may also be used for resistance to strengthen less affected muscles. The benefit of aquatic therapy is that many muscles can be worked at the same time. Individuals with a wide range of disabilities can participate in and enjoy aquatic therapy.

Aquatic therapy
A therapeutic regimen that is conducted in a pool, so that the water can support the body while also providing resistance to work muscles.

There are many other goals of PT, for example, to support optimal heart and lung function, optimize energy efficiency and conservation, and prevent and minimize pain. Physical therapists also provide fall risk assessment and develop individualized prevention strategies. They teach caregivers proper stretching, handling, and transfer techniques. Physical therapists also help determine the best **adaptive devices and equipment** as individuals lose function. Overall PT supports functional independence and participation in school, work, and the community and optimizes quality of life.

Adaptive devices and equipment
Wheelchairs and other devices used to assist disabled persons in mobility or other daily functions.

With all those potential benefits, it is illogical that many insurance companies do not cover continued PT. It is important to work with your interdisciplinary team to identify specific goals to be attained through PT and present this information to the insurance company. Strong letters of medical necessity are often needed to get this highly beneficial service.

Tayjus' Comment:

With DMD, PT is critical from diagnosis. It is so important to help maintain function. PT also helps make it possible for us to be independent longer and be able to carry out our ADLs. I have always enjoyed PT both at home and school, even becoming great friends with physical therapists. I have found that I feel better and am less afraid to be moved whether that is for dressing or traveling. As a kid, my parents used to do a lot of PT at home, but this was harder as I got busy with school. In college, however, I did make sure that I was able to have PT at least once a week. One challenge has been finding either a physical therapist who can come to your home or one who has a Hoyer lift in the facility. Overall, I think that it is crucial that everyone with MD receive PT from diagnosis.

Vicky's Comment:

The pool is the one place my son's body is free to stretch and move. Initially, he would boast that he could "walk" in the water. As his muscles weakened and he found it difficult to pick up his head from the water, we started using a snorkel, which helped immensely. He could swim laps at a time without having to lift his head out of the water. His doctors and I strongly believe that aquatic therapy has contributed to his healthy heart and lungs. Being a real foodie, it is an excellent way to burn calories and get some exercise.

Lilleen's Comment:

Physical therapy is important for those living with MD to keep your muscles strong for as long as you can. However, you should realize that what works for one person may not work for another. Therefore, you must work with your physical therapist to help him or her understand what your needs are and what you can or can't do. There are several ways to stay active through PT. I have found that aquatic therapy has been the most rewarding. The things I normally could not do on land, I can do in the water.

Colin's Comment:

I have had extensive experience with PT, both to aid in recovery from an injury and to manage the progression of my MD. It was necessary for me to try out different providers to find the best fit. I tried PT associated with a hospital and also a private practice. I usually went to receive PT at the office, but once or twice I received it at home when I was too injured to travel. I think that the benefits from PT are myriad, and my personal experience with it has been very positive. It has helped me with comfort and mobility and my physical therapist developed a plan that enabled me to dance at my sister's wedding. Although it can be challenging to find the right physical therapist for your situation. I think that people with any form of MD can benefit from regular PT.

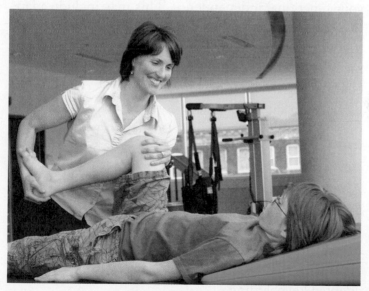

Figure 4 A physical therapist stretching leg muscles of a boy with FSHD.

19. What is occupational therapy?

Occupational therapy (OT) promotes health and well-being through ADLs or "occupations." These include schoolwork, housework, leisure activities, work-related activities, and personal care tasks such as dressing, bathing, or toileting. Occupational therapists help individuals be as independent as possible carrying out these activities by teaching new skills or adaptations to improve quality of life.

Similar to your appointment with a physical therapist, your appointment with an occupational therapist begins with an assessment of your current function and needs. This assessment may be done at an interdisciplinary clinic visit, an outpatient therapy appointment, school, or home. It will include an assessment of your safety and what assistive devices you are using.

After assessing your needs, the occupational therapist may recommend techniques or equipment to maximize your functional independence. This may include adaptive strategies for eating, grooming, dressing, bathing, toileting, or mobility. Equipment recommendations may include, for example, commode chairs, shower chairs, hospital bed, or Hoyer lift. The occupational therapist evaluates the need for a mobility device and may conduct a seating clinic evaluation where you are fitted for a scooter or wheelchair (power or manual).

An occupational therapist may make recommendations for home, school, or workplace adaptations, including ramps, bathroom alterations, and door alterations. He or she can advise teachers on alternative ways for the child with MD to perform schoolwork from scribes to adapted keyboarding.

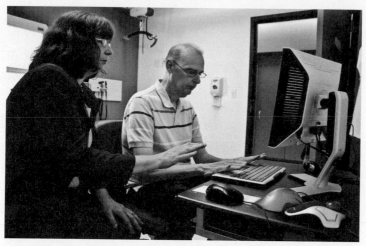

Figure 5 An occupational therapist introducing different mouse and keyboard options to an individual with DM1.

There is some overlap between what your physical therapist can do and what your occupational therapist can do for you. Physical therapists are generally concerned about gross motor movements. Occupational therapists are more focused on fine motor movements and therefore the hands (see **Figure 5**). OTs prescribe arm, wrist, and hand range-of-motion and gentle strengthening exercises. They may suggest or fashion resting hand splints to maintain wrist and finger range of motion.

OT is beneficial throughout the life span of those with MD, increasing independence and improving quality of life.

Tayjus' Comment:

All through school, from first through twelfth grade, I saw an occupational therapist regularly at school. I actually found the arm and hand stretches they would do with me the most helpful. I would work on fine motor skills through exercises like picking up coins in one hand and using putty.

I have also worked closely with occupational therapists in seating clinics. An occupational therapist can definitely be very useful to help someone with MD figure out how to do things differently and are definitely critical for trying to maintain independent living and occupational function.

Lilleen's Comment:

Working with an occupational therapist doesn't always mean gadgets or tools. For me, it was how to better arrange the furniture in my home for safer and better flow path and how to rearrange my kitchen for better accessibility to the items I used more often. For my son, his occupational therapist was able to show him ways he could take notes in class with a special pen that recorded while he wrote. Later, in high school, he used an iPad to type notes and record.

20. Are supplements for muscles effective and safe to take?

It is tempting to try various different supplements in the hopes that they provide a benefit to muscle. However, it is worth remembering that there are very few data to support the use of supplements in MD, and there can be risks of unintended side effects. I will discuss a few supplements that appear safe in moderation.

Creatine is essential to energy metabolism. It appears to increase energy availability and improve the formation of new muscle fibers from precursor cells. Creatine has a well-known capability to increase muscle strength in athletes and bodybuilders. Its effects in MD are less clear. Some studies have reported improvement in function while others have not. A Cochrane meta-analysis (combining data of multiple studies) of creatine in MD revealed a significant increase in muscle strength in the creatine-treated group compared to placebo.[5] Importantly, none of these studies reported side effects to creatine. Creatine monohydrate is safe at doses up to 5 grams a day for children and 10 grams a day for adults with the exception of those who have poor kidney function.

Coenzyme Q10 (CoQ10) or ubiquinone is found in the muscle mitochondria, the powerhouse of the cell, where it is crucial for energy metabolism. CoQ10 can also function as an antioxidant. CoQ10 levels may be low in some MDs such as DMD, BMD, and DM. One small study of CoQ10 in DMD was suggestive of a positive effect.[6] CoQ10 is safe at doses up to 300 mg a day in children and 900 mg a day in adults.

L-arginine and its precursor, *L-citrulline*, are important in the production of a chemical messenger, nitric oxide (NO). NO is low in MDs such as DMD, BMD, and some LGMD. Boosting NO levels through L-arginine or L-citrulline has the potential to improve mitochondrial function and blood flow. In a small trial of L-arginine and metformin (a drug that lowers blood glucose levels and that may also have effects on NO) in DMD, there was evidence of increased NO production and improved muscle function.[7] At the time of this publication, there is a current clinical trial of L-citrulline and metformin in DMD. L-arginine and L-citrulline are safe at doses of 2.5 grams three times daily.

Green tea extract has antioxidant and anti-inflammatory properties. There have been no trials of green tea extract in muscular dystrophy. In athletes, green tea extract reduces CK levels (a measure of muscle breakdown) and markers of oxidative stress. Green tea extract was generally found to be safe and well tolerated, although at high doses can cause liver toxicity. There is large variability in the composition of different green tea extract preparations—for example, you may not get the same amount of active ingredient if the green tea is taken as a beverage versus a capsule. The dose of epigallocatechin gallate (EGCG), an ingredient in green tea, is key to determining potential toxicity. An EGCG dose of 704 mg a day in beverage form or 338 mg a day in solid form has been shown to be safe in adults.[8]

For information about taking calcium and vitamin D supplements for bone health see Questions 48 and 56.

These are just a few of a myriad of supplements that are on the market for muscle health. Other supplements were not covered in this answer because there is insufficient data in humans to recommend their safety. It is worth remembering that supplements are not regulated by the FDA. This means that the amount of active agent may vary between preparations and brands. There may also be traces of impurities, such as a heavy metals, that can be harmful. You should talk to your doctor before starting on any supplement for MD.

21. Do corticosteroids help?

Corticosteroids are a class of synthetic drugs that are similar to the natural hormone cortisol produced by the adrenal glands. They include drugs such as prednisone, prednisolone, and deflazacort. The benefit of corticosteroids depends on the specific MD diagnosis. For most MDs, we simply don't have enough data to know if they would be helpful. For some MDs, such as LGMD 2B, corticosteroids appear to be harmful. Due to the numerous side effects of corticosteroids, the risks likely outweigh the benefits in adult-onset MD.

There is one MD for which we do have a lot of data on corticosteroids, and that is DMD. Corticosteroids prolong walking by as much as 3 years and also prolong arm functions such as the ability to feed oneself by as much as 2 years in DMD. The Centers for Disease Control and Prevention has issued guidelines to physicians and families on the treatment of DMD and recommends beginning corticosteroids before the phase of decline in function (typically age 6–8).[1] The guidelines also recommend continuing corticosteroids after the child loses ambulation for the positive effects they may have on arm muscles and muscles of respiration. Typical starting doses are 0.75 mg/kg/day for prednisone and 0.9 mg/kg/day deflazacort.

Unfortunately, there are many side effects of corticosteroids. The three major side effects are weight gain, bone fragility, and mood disturbance. There are a host of other potential consequences to chronic corticosteroid use including cataracts, delayed puberty, and short stature. These side effects frequently limit the amount of corticosteroids an adolescent or adult is on, which is typically lower in milligrams per kilogram than the starting dose. In the setting of intolerable side effects, the recommendation is to try an alternative dosing regimen such as weekend-only dosing, or to drop the total dose by one-third.

When taking corticosteroids chronically, the natural ability of the adrenal glands to produce steroids becomes suppressed. This has some important ramifications. It is important not to abruptly stop corticosteroids; they must be tapered slowly. If a child is vomiting and can't keep down his daily dose, it is necessary to deliver it intramuscularly (IM) or intravenously (IV), and every family should have a prescription for solucortef IM. Finally, in the event of a serious illness, surgery, or trauma the child may need "stress dose steroids," which are larger doses of steroids to overcome the adrenal insufficiency.

All of that sounds scary, but corticosteroids can be safely given to boys with DMD who reap the benefit of prolonged muscle function. So yes, corticosteroids help in the setting of DMD but probably don't in adult-onset MD.

Tayjus' Comment:

I would say I definitely have a love-hate relationship with corticosteroids. I have been taking them since the age of 5 or 6, so like many other boys with DMD, I have been taking corticosteroids for much of my life. When I first started taking steroids, I immediately gained a lot of weight and became quite chubby. My parents knew that they had to change our diet, so we got rid of junk food in our house and started eating a lot healthier. By high school, it also became clear that my puberty was delayed. Classmates and friends had much deeper voices and facial hair. Back in high school, looking much younger never bothered me, but in college, it really did start to bother me. I think looking so young and being in a wheelchair made people (outside of college and my friends) assume that I had some cognitive delays. I always wondered if people would even listen to me or if it was affecting internship and job interviews. But through all of this, I think I have always felt that steroids have been beneficial. They have kept me walking longer, they have delayed the speed of progression, and I believe they are maintaining my pulmonary and cardiac function. As for the many annoying side effects, many of them can be addressed. As many boys with DMD will tell you, the biggest frustration is that we look so much younger. But steroids have also kept many of us healthier.

22. Does testosterone make muscle stronger?

Testosterone is an androgen and anabolic steroid. Androgens stimulate the development of male sex characteristics. Anabolic steroids promote lean muscle mass and strength. There is widespread use and abuse of testosterone by bodybuilders and athletes seeking to improve performance and muscle mass. So could it also be helpful to individuals with MD?

There have been relatively few studies of testosterone in MD. What we do know is that testosterone levels decrease in men with aging and as a side effect of some conditions and treatments, leading to reduced lean muscle mass, low muscle strength, and predisposition to falls. Testosterone replacement in these scenarios of hypogonadal healthy men (men in whom the testes are not producing enough testosterone) increases fat-free muscle mass and strength. It is less clear in MD individuals. In a clinical trial, testosterone given to men with DM increased muscle mass but not muscle strength.[9] In another clinical trial, an oral synthetic analog of testosterone, oxandrolone in DMD increased strength by some measures but not by others.[10] At the time of this publication, there is an ongoing study of testosterone and human growth hormone in FSHD.

While it is unclear if testosterone makes muscle stronger in MD individuals, there are other advantages of testosterone for some men and adolescent boys. (Due to the masculinization induced by testosterone, it is not considered medically appropriate for women.) Many men with DM and boys with DMD are hypogonadal, either because of the disease itself or because of medications used. Specifically, corticosteroids such as prednisone may inhibit and/or delay puberty. The delay in puberty has implications for bone strength, growth, energy, psychological development, and sexual function. Bone mass typically increases by 50% during normal puberty. Androgen deficiency is a recognized factor for osteoporosis and fracture and androgen replacement therapy is associated with improved bone density. It may also increase energy and sexual function in men. Testosterone replacement will lead to the development of puberty and may increase bone density and vertical growth.

Testosterone comes in several different formulations including intramuscular injections and topical preparations. There are potential side effects to testosterone therapy including for boys: emotional lability, acne, body odor, and epiphyseal closure (closure of the growth plates resulting in the end of vertical growth). In addition, for adults there is increased risk of prostate hypertrophy, potentially prostate cancer (although this risk is unclear), breast development with swelling or tenderness, blood clots, heart attack, and stroke. Despite these potential side effects, testosterone is generally well tolerated and considered to be beneficial in hypogonadal men and boys.

If you are a man with MD, you may wish to have a testosterone level checked by your neurologist, internist, or endocrinologist. It is important that this blood test be done in the early morning when testosterone levels peak. For boys with MD, absence of pubertal development by age 14 should precipitate a referral to an endocrinologist.

Tayjus' Comment:

When I was around 14, I started taking testosterone partly so that I would start to look my age, but also for the benefit of bone health. I still take testosterone today and I have tried it in the form of an ointment, a patch, and a shot every two weeks, which I prefer. I think for the most part it has been helpful. It is clear that puberty is delayed for most boys on steroids. It is still frustrating being mistaken for a high schooler or being called "ma'am" on the phone. Overall, I think I am glad I started on testosterone, but of course like with many teens it can make me more moody. But in the long run, I do think it is good that I have been taking it both for my physical health including bone health as well for my general happiness. At the end of the day we are just like anyone else and we want to be treated as normally as possible.

Colin's Comment:

In my late 20s, a blood test revealed low levels of testosterone. My neurologist recommended testosterone replacement therapy. I have been using the patches ever since. I immediately noticed a change in my energy level. While I don't really have any of what most people would consider energy, using the patches brought my energy level from nonexistent to low. I still don't have a lot of energy, but at least I have some. Those around me noticed a difference too. I didn't notice any serious side effects of taking the testosterone and the only complaints I have are specific to using the patches, but they are the delivery systems that work the best for me. Overall, I found that the testosterone replacement therapy was helpful.

23. What about bracing?

A brace may be prescribed for muscle weakness or contracture (shortening of tendon). There are braces for many joints including ankles, knees, hands, and back.

Ankle foot orthoses (AFOs) are the most common braces used by those with MD. AFOs are for those who have weakness of muscles supporting the ankle and for those at risk of developing a contracture of the Achilles tendon that occurs when the muscles that push the foot down are much stronger than the muscles that pull the foot up.

Weak ankle muscles may make it difficult to pick up the foot to walk properly. This is called foot drop and can lead to tripping and falls. An AFO helps lift the foot and allows further walking without fatigue with less tripping and falling. AFOs for walking include custom-molded thermoplastic models and off-the-shelf carbon-fiber braces. For walking, many people prefer the carbon-fiber braces, which are lightweight and spring-like, reducing the energy cost of walking by replacing a substantial part of the ankle muscle work. However, other people will benefit from the increased lateral stability that the custom-molded thermoplastic models provide. It may take some time to get used to wearing AFOs, particularly while driving and walking downhill. You many need to find new shoes to accommodate the AFOs.

Ankle foot orthoses (AFOs)

A type of brace used in MD that supports the ankle and prevents contracture of the Achilles tendon.

Nighttime AFOs are prescribed for those who are at risk of developing contracture of the Achilles tendon. These should be custom-molded, thermoplastic AFOs. They may be nonarticulated AFOs with a fixed stiffness and joint or an articulated AFO that has a flexible mechanical joint, which allows repositioning of the ankle joint. Nighttime AFOs should be initiated soon after diagnosis for DMD and other similar childhood MDs at risk of developing contracture of the Achilles tendon. The child should not walk in them during the day, as this may throw off the child's balance. However, they can be worn when sitting—for example, while watching a movie or playing a video game. Combined with a daily stretching program, nighttime AFOs work to maintain the ankle joint in a neutral position. When initiated early in life, AFOs are generally well accepted and become part of the evening routine such as brushing teeth.

AFOs require a prescription from your doctor and fitting by a certified orthotist. AFOs should be comfortable, and it may take a few visits to the orthotist to get them just right. After that, you will likely be pleased with the benefit that they provide if you have ankle muscle weakness.

24. What are some general rules regarding stretching?

Some muscles are stronger than other muscles. When there is an imbalance of muscle strength across a joint, then shortening of the muscle, or contracture, can happen. An example of this is the biceps being stronger than the triceps, leading to a shortening of the biceps tendon and contracture at the elbow so that it cannot be fully straightened. Another common example is the muscles that point the foot, gastrocnemius and soleus, being stronger than the muscles that flex the foot, tibialis anterior. This leads to shortening of the Achilles tendon and toe walking. Moderate to severe contractures can lead to a decrease in motor function. Luckily, something can be done about these contractures: you can stretch.

Stretching should be a regular part of everyday care of a person with MD who has muscle tightness or contractures. When the person is a young child, the stretching is usually done by an adult, such as the parent. When older, the level of involvement of a parent or physical therapist depends on the level of weakness. For example, an older child with DMD or an adult with adult-onset MD may be able to stand on a wedge or lean against the wall to stretch the Achilles.

The muscles that are stretched each day depend on which ones are tight and developing contractures. For example, in the young boy with DMD, stretching involves the ankles, knees, and hips. In older individuals with DMD, the emphasis turns to the forearms, wrists, and fingers, as these are crucial for continued abilities such as driving a wheelchair and operating a computer. A physical therapist should evaluate the individual with MD at least twice each year for DMD, and at least once each year for adult MD, to make recommendations on which muscles to stretch. The physical therapist will also give instructions on the best techniques for stretching. Parent Project Muscular Dystrophy (PPMD) has an excellent YouTube video that describes several stretches for a boy with DMD (https://www.youtube.com/watch?v=0_ecVd3kNtQ).

Some general rules of stretching include:

1. **Proper positioning** for each stretching activity is crucial. Refer to instructions provided by your physical therapist.
2. **Stabilize** the joints not being stretched. These include joints above or below the joint being stretched.
3. Stretching should not be painful. Overstretching may be detrimental to muscle health.
4. Do not stretch against resistance. It is important that the individual relaxes.
5. Stretching of each muscle should last for a count of 30, repeated three times. The whole sequence of stretching all muscles need only last 10–15 minutes a day.

Stretching is one of the ways in which an individual and family can be proactive in the fight against MD. It is an investment that is every bit worth the effort.

Vicky's Comment:

If there was one thing I'd encourage parents to give the highest priority in caring for a Duchenne boy, it's daily stretching. My son benefited greatly from hip, hamstring and Achilles stretches when he was ambulatory. We made the mistake of reducing the stretching after he stopped walking, and very quickly, we saw contractures develop in his hips and ankles. Once contractures develop, they're difficult to reverse.

References

1. Voet NBM, et al. Strength training and aerobic exercise training for muscle disease. *Cochrane Database of Systematic Reviews* 2013;7.

2. Tawil R, et al. Evidence-based guideline summary: Evaluation, diagnosis, and management of facioscapulohumeral muscular dystrophy. Report of the Guideline Development, Dissemination, and Implementation Subcommittee of the American Academy of Neurology and the Practice Issues Review Panel of the American Association of Neuromuscular & Electrodiagnostic Medicine. *Neurology* 2015;85(4):357–364.

3. Ashizawa T, et al. Consensus-based care recommendations for adults with myotonic dystrophy type 1. *Neurology Clinical Practice* 2018;8(6):507–520.

4. Case LE, et al. Rehabilitative management of the patient with Duchenne muscular dystrophy. *Pediatrics* 2018;142(s2): S17–S33.

5. Kley RA, Tarnopolsky MA, Vorgerd M. Creatine for treating muscle disorders. *Cochrane Database Systematic Reviews* 2013; 6: CD004760. https://doi.org/10.1002/14651858.CD004760 .pub4

6. Spurney CF, et al. CINRG pilot trial of coenzyme Q10 in steroid-treated Duchenne muscular dystrophy. *Muscle Nerve* 2011;44:174–178.

7. Hafner P, et al. Improved muscle function in Duchenne muscular dystrophy through L-arginine and metformin: An investigator-initiated, open-label, single-center, proof-of-concept study. *PLoS One* 2016;11(1):e0147634.

8. Hu J, et al. The safety of green tea and green tea extract consumption in adults—Results of a systematic review. *Regulatory Toxicology and Pharmacology* 2018;95:412–433.

9. Birnkrant DJ, Bushby K, Bann CM, Apkon SD, Blackwell A, Brumbaugh D, Case LE, Clemens PR, Hadiyannakis S, Pandya S, Street N, Tomezsko J, Wagner KR, Ward LM, Weber DR for the DMD Care Considerations Working Group. Diagnosis and management of Duchenne muscular dystrophy, part 1: diagnosis, and neuromuscular, rehabilitation, endocrine, and gastrointestinal and nutritional management. *Lancet Neurology* 2018;17(3):251–267.

10. Griggs RC, et al. Randomized controlled trial of testosterone in myotonic dystrophy. *Neurology* 1989;39:219–222.

11. Fenichel GM, et al. A randomized efficacy and safety trial of oxandrolone in the treatment of Duchenne dystrophy. *Neurology* 2001;56:1075–1079.

New Therapeutic Options

What is gene therapy?

What is genome editing?

What is a clinical trial?

More . . .

25. What is exon skipping?

Exon skipping is a relatively new approach to treating genetic disorders and is currently being developed for DMD. Exons are the portion of our DNA that code for proteins. A gene is made up of multiple exons that are separated by noncoding DNA called **introns**. The *DMD* gene, for example, is made up of 79 exons (see **Figure 6**). This gene provides the instructions to make a protein called dystrophin. Genetic changes that result in loss of dystrophin cause DMD. Inside our cells, the DNA message is "read" to make the protein, but first, the introns must be taken out of the message so that the exons join together. You can see in the figure that the exons fit together like pieces of a puzzle. The most common type of genetic change causing DMD is a deletion. For individuals with certain deletions, the

Intron

A segment of a gene that does not code for a protein.

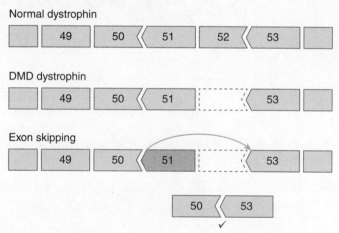

Figure 6 Diagram of exon skipping. Normal dystrophin has 79 exons; a portion of the gene is shown here, where exons are in gray, and introns are in white. In the accompanying example of DMD dystrophin, exon 52 is missing; there are hundreds of other possible mutations in the dystrophin gene, but this is just one. In exon skipping, an ASO is given to cause the cell to skip over an additional exon, here exon 51, to restore dystrophin expression.

cell cannot make dystrophin because the reading of the gene is "out of frame." For example, if you had a deletion of exon 52 in the *DMD* gene, you can see that exon 51 does not fit with exon 53, and therefore no dystrophin would be made.

Researchers have discovered that if you give a small piece of nucleic acid, called an antisense oligonucleotide (ASO), that binds to the region where the intron and exon meet, you can induce the cell to skip over an exon. If you skip over exon 51, you can see that exon 50 now fits with exon 53, and the reading of the gene is back in frame, and you make dystrophin (although with a small piece missing in the middle). It is known that if there is some dystrophin, even with a small piece missing, the MD is less severe—as it is in BMD.

The first exon-skipping drug for MD to be approved by the U.S. Food and Drug Administration (FDA) was eteplirsen (Exondys 51) for DMD. This drug is appropriate for approximately 13% of those with DMD— those in whom skipping exon 51 would put their gene back in frame. Eteplirsen was granted accelerated approval by the FDA. The second exon-skipping drug for MD to be approved was golodirsen (Vyondys 53) for DMD. This drug is appropriate for approximately 8% of those with DMD, those patients who would benefit from skipping exon 53. Also in development are ASOs that are aimed at skipping exon 45. Approximately 60–80% of all DMD patients have mutations that would be amenable to some form of exon skipping. Your neurologist and genetic counselor can help you determine if you or your son's mutation is amenable to eterplirsen, golodirsen, or another drug in development that skips a different exon.

ASOs are administered through an intravenous infusion. Most current ASOs are given on a weekly basis. To avoid having to endure frequent needlesticks to start a peripheral IV for the infusion, many patients choose to have a **port-a-cath** placed. This is a device that is placed under the skin in the chest that is connected to a catheter or small tube that is inserted into the superior vena cava, which is the large blood vessel that enters into the top right chamber of the heart. The infusion can then occur via the port, which is the entry point for the infusion needle. A port is only visible as a small lump under the skin. Ports have the advantage of avoiding frequent needlesticks and bruising. They also come with some risks, such as infection, blockage, and clots.

There is quite a lot of activity in the field of exon skipping. While two drugs for exon skipping have already been approved, others are in clinical trials, including newer generations of ASOs that may be more efficacious.

26. What is gene therapy?

Gene therapy is the addition, subtraction, or change in genetic material in the cells of an individual who is being treated for a disease. Many of the MDs are caused by a faulty gene that leads to an absent protein. In these cases, gene therapy aims to introduce a version of the gene to enable the cell to make a functional protein. Other MDs are caused by the abnormal expression of a gene that leads to a toxic RNA or protein. In these cases, gene therapy aims to silence the gene—that is, to prevent it from making the RNA or protein.

Port-a-cath

A device set under a patient's skin that combines a port (opening) and a catheter (tube), allowing IV medications to be infused directly into a vein so the patient doesn't have to endure multiple needlesticks.

Gene therapy

The addition, subtraction, or change in genetic material in the cells of an individual who is being treated for a disease.

Gene therapy takes advantage of viruses (vectors) that can deliver genetic material to the cells of the individual. These viruses have been gutted of their own genes and cannot cause disease. The vector that is most commonly used is adeno-associated virus (AAV). The new genetic material is packaged in the AAV, which then delivers it to the inside of the cell. Inside the cell, the new genetic material does not integrate into the patient's genes, where it might cause problems, but remains separate in the cell.

There is quite a bit of excitement about gene therapy now that the first gene therapies for retinal dystrophy and spinal muscular atrophy have been FDA approved. Gene therapies for DMD and LGMD2E are in clinical trials, and gene therepies for DM, FSHD, LGMD2A, LGMD2B, and LGMD2I are in development.

Currently, in clinical trials for MD, AAV is being given to individuals through an intravenous infusion. This allows all of the muscles of the body to be treated. From animal studies and gene therapy studies in other diseases, it is believed that the new genetic material will be expressed for a number of years. It will not likely be expressed for the life of the individual because of the fact that it is anticipated that there will still be some turnover of muscle during which the new genetic material will be lost. So, gene therapy may not be a one-time treatment, but should be effective for several years.

Gene therapy will likely not cure MD, but has the potential to be a very effective treatment. In some cases, such as for DMD, only a smaller version of the faulty gene (in this case dystrophin) can be packaged into AAV—and this smaller version is not fully functional. It is also possible that gene therapy will not generate as much expression of the required genetic material as exists in normal individuals. As described above, the effects of gene therapy are expected to wane over time. Finally, muscle that has already been converted to fat and scar tissue (fibrosis), would not be amenable to gene therapy and so functions that have been lost may not be recoverable.

There are risks to gene therapy. Unlike other treatments, you can't stop it once given. The body may mount an immune response to the vector, which may result in injury to other organs. It is even possible that the body may mount an immune response to the new protein being expressed, which it may identify as being "foreign."

Currently to qualify for gene therapy, it is important that you do not have preexisting antibodies to AAV. These could reduce the effectiveness of the gene therapy or lead to significant safety issues. A substantial proportion of the population has been exposed to AAV and has antibodies. Research is under way to figure out how to deliver gene therapy to those with antibodies. This is also an important challenge to overcome in order to re-dose individuals who become immunized against AAV with their first treatment.

The field of gene therapy is moving very quickly, and it is likely that we will be able to overcome challenges such as preexisting antibodies and redosing in the near future. Gene therapy holds the promise of providing a truly meaningful treatment for many of the MDs in which there are few other therapeutic options.

27. *What is genome editing?*

Genome editing is a relatively new technology that allows scientists to add, subtract, or alter the DNA in an organism's living cells. In the past, scientists could only manipulate DNA if it were out of the body. After they made changes, they could put it back into the body using a delivery vehicle, such as a virus. This latter example is commonly referred to as "gene therapy," which is an approach to deliver genetic material to a cell, as described in Question 26. In contrast, gene editing directly changes the genes already in the cells. Genome editing makes a permanent change in the cell's DNA. It does this through a molecular scissors that cuts the DNA at a specific sequence. When the cell repairs the cut, a change is made in the sequence. This provides an opportunity to remove the gene (for those with dominantly inherited MD), remove one or more exons (similar to exon skipping; see Question 25), or to correct a small underlying mutation causing the disease.

Genome editing

A procedure that makes permanent changes in the DNA of a living cell in the body.

Genome editing has been greatly enhanced by the discovery of the Clustered Regularly Interspaced Short Palindromic Repeats (CRISPR)/Cas9 system. This is a bacteria-derived system that efficiently targets a specific sequence of DNA and makes a cut. Genome editing is sometimes referred to as **CRISPR** for this reason.

CRISPR

A recently discovered method of genome editing derived from bacteria that targets a specific DNA sequence and modifies it.

Genome editing has shown promise in mouse and dog models of MD. There are still challenges that need to be overcome before this technology is used for human patients with MD. This includes ensuring that the technology is safe (that the cuts to the DNA do not occur in the wrong regions), minimizing an immune response to the bacteria-derived portions of the system, and maximizing the efficiency of the editing to occur in all muscle cells. Currently the CRISPR/Cas9 system is delivered to cells through AAV and thus has some of the same limitations that gene therapy has, including the problem of preexisting neutralizing antibodies.

28. What are stem cells?

Stem cells

Unspecialized cells that have the ability both to renew themselves and to differentiate into specific types of cells in the body.

Differentiation

The process in which a stem cell develops into a more specific type of cell, such as a blood or muscle cell.

Pluripotent

Capable of giving rise to several different types of specialized cell types.

Satellite cell

An adult stem cell found in skeletal muscle that can replicate and differentiate into new muscle fibers.

Stem cells have several unique characteristics that set them apart from other cells and provide a future promise for the understanding and treatment of MD. Stem cells have the ability to replicate and renew themselves. They are unspecialized cells, meaning that they do not have the characteristics and function of cells of specific tissues and organs such as nerve, cardiac, or skin cells. However, they have the ability to give rise to a variety of specialized cells in a process called **differentiation**. A stem cell capable of differentiating into several different specialized cell types is called **pluripotent**.

There are different types of stem cells. Embryonic stem cells come from embryos at the 3–5 cell stage and are pluripotent, capable of developing into any cell type. Human embryonic stem cells come from unused embryos left over from in vitro fertilization obtained with informed consent. The U.S. government prohibits the use of federal funds for research using human embryonic stem cells not currently listed in a registry.

Adult stem cells come from fully developed tissues. These cells develop into only a limited number of other cell types. In skeletal muscle, the adult stem cell is called the **satellite cell**. Satellite cells lie dormant in muscle until they are activated to replicate and differentiate, after which they form new muscle fibers. There were clinical trials of transplantation of satellite cells into individuals with MD in the 1980s that did not show substantial survival of transplanted cells. One problem with adult stem cells is that there are small numbers of them in any given tissue and it is difficult to expand their numbers in the lab. Another problem is that the body may recognize the adult stem cell from a donor as foreign and mount an immune response against it.

Induced pluripotent stem cells (iPSCs) are adult stem cells that have been manipulated in the laboratory to become pluripotent like embryonic stem cells. iPSCs can be derived from skin cells and differentiated into muscle cells. There is therefore hope that one could make new muscle cells for an individual beginning with his or her own cells, thus bypassing the immune response. In the laboratory, one can also correct the disease gene in iPSCs, thus allowing for transplantation of healthy new muscle cells. Although transplantation of iPSC-derived muscle cells is still several years away from clinical trials, iPSCs are currently being used for drug screens and disease modeling for MD.

Induced pluripotent stem cells (iPSCs)

Adult stem cells that have been manipulated in the laboratory to become pluripotent like embryonic stem cells.

Perinatal stem cells include those found in amniotic fluid and umbilical cord blood. Stem cells from umbilical cord blood can be banked for future use without harm to the baby. This is an expensive procedure, and there are currently no treatments for MD using umbilical cord stem cells. However, such stem cells would not trigger an immune response if given back to the same individual. More research is needed on development of umbilical cord stem cells for therapy.

Stem cells hold great promise for the future for regenerating muscle. However, throughout the world, there are clinics advertising "stem cell therapy." It is important to recognize that most of these do not have regulatory approval (such as from the FDA) and do not have the science behind them to justify being called a treatment. Many are illegal, and the treatments they provide may have no effect or may even be dangerous. Before participating in any "stem cell therapy," check with your healthcare providers.

29. What is a clinical trial?

Clinical trial

A research study in human volunteers that is designed to test the safety and/or efficacy of an intervention.

Preclinical studies

Research performed on a new drug prior to entry into human clinical trials.

Protocol

The research plan that describes which individuals are eligible to participate in the trial, what drugs are used and at which dosages, the tests and measures to be performed, and the schedule and duration of the study.

A **clinical trial** is a research study in human volunteers that is designed to test the safety and/or efficacy of an intervention. This intervention may be a new drug or device or a new use for a drug already approved by the FDA. Clinical trials in humans follow "preclinical" studies in animals. **Preclinical studies** aim to establish that the drug is effective in an animal model of disease and determine potential toxic effects at various doses. Preclinical studies also help to answer questions about drug absorption, metabolism, and elimination.

Clinical trials adhere to a specific plan or **protocol** that dictates which individuals are eligible to participate in the trial, the drugs and dosages, the tests and measures that will be performed, the study schedule and the length of the study. The protocol is reviewed and approved by an Institutional Review Board (IRB), which safeguards the rights and the welfare of the individuals participating in the trial.

Clinical trials are conducted in phases. Each phase has different objectives, risks, and potential benefits. Phase 1 trials are the first trials of a new drug in a small number of human volunteers. Volunteers may be healthy or may have the targeted disease. These trials aim to determine what is a safe and tolerable dose of drug to administer and what potential **side effects** of the drug are present. Phase 1 trials also provide information about how the drug is processed in the body. These trials are usually short in duration. Phase 1 trials are often designed so that small groups of volunteers (e.g., 3 to 6 individuals) receive one of a predefined dose level. Doses are initially very low and are based on the toxicology data from the preclinical studies. Trials may begin as a Single Ascending Dose (SAD) trial in which volunteers receive a single dose of the drug, then monitored for their response to it. After a dose level is found to be safe, then the next group of volunteers receives a higher single dose. This continues until a predetermined safety threshold is reached or until intolerable side effects are observed. A SAD trial may be followed by a Multiple Ascending Dose (MAD) trial, in which volunteers receive multiple doses of the drug for a defined period of time. Again, after a dose level is found to be safe, then the next group of volunteers receives multiple doses of a higher dose level. A committee of experts called the Data and Safety Monitoring Board (DSMB) evaluates the safety of the new drug and approves the increase in dose level. Phase 1 trials expose the volunteer to risk with little potential for benefit due to the short duration of the trial and low doses administered. However, phase 1 trials in MD are often coupled to Open Label Extension (OLE) studies in which all participants are allowed to continue on the maximum tolerated dose. During the OLE, volunteers may have the potential to benefit from receiving the drug over a longer period of time.

Phase 2 trials are designed to continue to provide safety information and to determine efficacy of the drug. These trials are in larger numbers of human volunteers (e.g., 20–300 individuals) who have the targeted disease but

Side effects
Effects of a treatment that are not the ones intended to treat the disease.

are restricted to volunteers with defined characteristics. Phase 2 trials are usually randomized and controlled. This means that volunteers are randomly assigned to receive either the drug or a **placebo** (a sham or inactive product that resembles the drug). Phase 2 trials are also frequently **double-blinded**, meaning that neither the investigator nor the volunteer knows whether he or she is receiving drug or placebo. This reduces the risk of bias in the study. Phase 2 trials are sometimes divided into Phase 2A studies, which are specially designed to assess dosing, and Phase 2B studies, which are specially designed to determine efficacy. A Phase 2 trial may be followed by an OLE study so that the placebo group has the potential to benefit from the drug, too.

Phase 3 trials compare the new drug with the **standard of care**. The standard of care refers to a treatment that is routinely used in day-to-day clinical practice. For example, corticosteroids are the standard of care for DMD. Phase 3 trials typically require even larger numbers of volunteers in order to demonstrate that the study drug is "noninferior" to the standard of care. A Phase 3 trial may be designed to expand the patient population targeted.

Phase 4 trials are conducted after the new drug has received approval from the FDA. These trials are for "postmarketing surveillance." They provide information on the safety of the drug in large populations, highlighting side effects that may not have been seen in the limited number of subjects in Phase 1–3 trials. They also provide information on the long-term safety of the drug. Under these circumstances, less common side effects may be detected.

There are risks to participating in a clinical trial. You may have side effects from the drug that are unpleasant,

Placebo

A sham or inactive product that resembles the drug, given to volunteers in a clinical trial as a way of determining a treatment effect.

Double-blinded

A research trial in which neither the volunteer nor the researchers know whether the volunteer was given the actual treatment or the placebo until the end in order to avoid bias.

Standard of care

A treatment that is routinely used in day-to-day clinical practice in patients with the disease being investigated.

serious, or even life-threatening. You may have adverse effects from the testing such as from muscle biopsy (see Question 32), blood testing, or muscle function testing. You will need to make frequent visits to the medical center, likely causing you to miss school or work.

Despite these risks, there are many reasons why you might want to participate in a clinical trial. These include the ability to move the field forward by helping establish the safety and efficacy of a new treatment and provide a benefit to others with the same disease. There is also the possibility that you will directly benefit from a new drug before it is FDA approved. Finally, you may benefit from the enhanced medical attention that you receive during the trial. Participation in a clinical trial can be very rewarding.

30. How do I find a clinical trial in which to participate?

Your neurologist and other healthcare providers are an excellent source of information to begin a search for a clinical trial. They may be participating in clinical trials and will have intimate knowledge of what is available to you at your medical center. They will also have a good sense as to whether you meet eligibility criteria (see Question 31). Finally, they may be familiar with the preclinical research on any trial you are considering and can help you understand the data supporting the trial.

Another great source of information is the website clinicaltrials.gov. This site is a service of the National Institutes of Health (NIH) and is maintained by the National Library of Medicine. Clinical trials of any FDA-regulated drug, biological, or device product other than phase 1 or small feasibility studies are required to register with clinicaltrials.gov. The website is easy to use. You can enter your condition, and all the applicable trials are displayed. You can then sort by "recruiting" status to find ones that are actively looking for volunteers. The website provides information on the design of the study, the arms of the trial (groups of participants that receive a specific intervention or no intervention), outcome measures (the ways in which the study will evaluate the effect of the intervention), eligibility criteria, the sponsor (who is responsible for initiating, managing, and financing the trial), and the investigators (who actually conducts the clinical trial, such as a neurologist). Once a trial is complete, the results of the trial are also listed on clinicaltrials.gov. A similar registry exists in the European Union: clinicaltrialsregister.eu.

Finally, many of the patient advocacy groups help advertise for clinical trials in MD. Through their websites and newsletters, you can be informed of actively recruiting clinical trials for your condition. See Appendix B for a list of patient advocacy groups for MD.

It is good to discuss your plans to participate in any clinical trial with your healthcare team. You may want their advice about whether to participate in any given trial, and you will certainly want them to know if you have enrolled in a clinical trial so that they can be informed of any potential adverse events or efficacy.

31. How do I qualify for a clinical trial?

Eligibility criteria

Rules about who can participate in a particular clinical trial.

Every clinical trial has rules about who can participate. These are called **eligibility criteria**. To be eligible for a particular clinical trial, the individual must have certain characteristics called inclusion criteria. In addition, the individual may not have certain qualities called exclusion criteria. These criteria include things such as specific genetic diagnosis, age, gender, health history, and functional abilities. The inclusion and exclusion criteria for all U.S. trials and many international trials can be found on the clincialtrials.gov website.

It can be frustrating and disappointing to be excluded from a clinical trial based on eligibility criteria. The purpose of having strict eligibility criteria is to ensure that all subjects are safe and to ensure that the results are accurate and meaningful. In this way, the trial has the greatest likelihood of success allowing the drug to go for regulatory approval and to become available to a wider population. After a drug is approved, it often becomes available to patients with many fewer restrictions than those required by clinical trials.

32. What's involved in a muscle biopsy?

If you participate in a clinical trial, you may be asked to have a **muscle biopsy**. Occasionally muscle biopsies are also used for diagnostic purposes. Small samples of muscle tissue can provide information about the health of the muscle, the expression of genes and proteins, and the distribution of drugs to muscle.

During a biopsy, a small amount of muscle tissue is taken from the belly of the muscle. The overall amount of tissue is insignificant compared to the overall size of the muscle and you will not be weaker from the procedure.

There are several different kinds of muscle biopsies. An open muscle biopsy is done in an operating room. Children are typically put to sleep for this procedure. Adults may receive some sedation and local anesthesia.

Muscle biopsy
Removal of a small amount of muscle tissue to gather information for diagnostic or clinical trial purposes.

After the skin over the muscle belly is cleaned, and local anesthesia is administered, an approximate 1-inch incision is made. The overlying fat and muscle covering (**fascia**) are separated, and the muscle is exposed. Several small strips of muscle the size of the top of a pencil eraser are taken. The fascia and skin are closed with dissolvable sutures, and a pressure bandage is applied. The individual is asked not to use the biopsied limb for a day and not to get the sutures wet for several days.

Fascia

Connective tissue lining of skeletal muscle.

Needle muscle biopsies are less invasive than open muscle biopsies. There are different size needles and techniques for these biopsies. Generally, these biopsies are done in an exam room and under local anesthesia. After cleaning the skin and infusing local anesthesia, a nick is made in the skin with a scalpel. A needle is passed through the opening in the skin, which retrieves a much smaller amount of tissue than in an open muscle biopsy. Sometimes, the doctor goes through the same opening several times with the needle in order to retrieve additional samples of muscle. Usually, needle muscle biopsies do not require sutures. A pressure bandage is applied. The individual can use the limb immediately, but should not submerge it in water for several days.

Muscle biopsies are relatively safe procedures. However, there are risks to muscle biopsy such as pain, bleeding, infection, nerve damage, formation of hematoma (collection of blood under the skin), or reaction to anesthesia. An open muscle biopsy will leave a scar.

You might ask why an open muscle biopsy is performed rather than a needle muscle biopsy if the latter is less invasive and doesn't leave a scar. The answer is that needle muscle biopsies do not always provide enough tissue to answer the question that is being asked in a clinical trial. Still, researchers are mindful of patient and family preferences, and needle muscle biopsies are being used more frequently when possible.

PART FIVE

Breathing

Should I get the influenza vaccine and other recommended vaccines?

What is spirometry?

When should I start using nighttime ventilatory support?

More . . .

33. Should I get the influenza vaccine and other recommended vaccines?

Yes! Influenza kills thousands of people and hospitalizes hundreds of thousands more each year. Influenza is especially deadly for those with chronic medical conditions or with respiratory conditions such as in MD. It can lead to pneumonia and **rhabdomyolysis** (massive breakdown of muscle tissue). The influenza vaccine does not guarantee that you will avoid the flu, but it does reduce the likelihood and also decrease the severity if you do get the flu. Because the strains of virus that cause flu change every year, it is important to get the annual vaccine each influenza season.

Influenza vaccines are safe. They do not cause the flu because they are inactivated (killed) or attenuated (weakened) viruses. They do not cause autism. They can cause some symptoms such as fever, muscle aches, or headache, but these usually dissipate in 1–2 days. This is the body's response to the vaccine, which will later protect you from a much more serious and potentially fatal infection.

People who are taking corticosteroids should opt for the inactivated influenza vaccine, which is an intramuscular shot, rather than the live, attenuated vaccine, which is a nasal spray. This is because corticosteroids may cause some degree of immunosuppression, and you could become ill from the live, attenuated vaccine.

Other important vaccines for respiratory health include the vaccines against *Streptococcus pneumoniae*, often called "pneumococcus," which can cause pneumonia and other serious diseases. There are two pneumococcal vaccines: Prevnar 13 (PCV13), which protects against

Rhabdomyolysis

Massive breakdown of muscle that can occur from exertion, infection, or certain anesthetic agents.

Because the strains of virus that cause flu change every year, it is important to get the annual vaccine each influenza season.

13 strains of the bacteria, and Pneumovax 23 (PPSV23), which protects against 23 strains. It is recommended that MD individuals over the age of 2 get both vaccines. These are both inactivated vaccines that are safe for those on corticosteroids to receive. Most people get vaccinated with Prevnar 13 as infants, and those with MD should then get one or two doses of Pneumovax 23 depending on whether they are immunosuppressed. If you didn't get vaccinated or don't know whether you were vaccinated with Prevnar 13 as an infant, then you will need to get this before your Pneumovax 23 shot. The vaccines last for several years. Complete recommendations for pneumococcal vaccination can be found on the CDC website https://www.cdc.gov/vaccines/schedules/hcp/imz/adult.html#note-pneumo.

You should remember that you may be immunosuppressed from chronic disease and/or use of corticosteroids. This may make you more susceptible to infections and illnesses. It is important to keep all your vaccines up to date and follow the vaccination schedule provided by your pediatrician or internist. Live attenuated vaccines such as MMR (measles, mumps, and rubella) and varicella (chickenpox) ideally should be given to children before they are started on corticosteroids. Keep a record of your vaccines and bring this record to your primary care physician and neurologist.

34. What is spirometry?

Spirometry is a simple test that your neurologist, pulmonologist, or respiratory therapist conducts with you in clinic to assess your breathing capacity. It is also known as a **pulmonary function test (PFT)**. During the test, you will be asked to put a mouthpiece in your

Pulmonary function test (PFT)

Different tests performed to assess how well your lungs and related muscles are working to keep oxygen coming in and carbon dioxide going out.

mouth or, if you have facial muscle weakness, to put on a mask, either of which are connected by a tube to the spirometer. A nose clip will be placed on your nose. Following several normal breaths, you will be asked to take as deep a breath in as you can and then let it out as fast and hard as you can, completely emptying your lungs. You will be asked to do this three times. The highest value from the three tests is considered the final result.

Spirometry provides several pieces of helpful information to your doctors. The **forced vital capacity (FVC)** is the measure of how much air you can exhale at full capacity. For MD, it is a measure of the diaphragm and other respiratory muscle strength. When FVC is low, this is referred to as a restrictive disorder of pulmonary function. The FVC correlates with the need for ventilator assistance such as BIPAP (see Question 37) and cough assistance (see Question 35). The **forced expiratory volume measured over 1 second (FEV1)** is a measure of how much air can be expelled in the first second of exhalation. FEV1/FVC gives the proportion of air that can be expelled from the individual's lungs in the first second. FEV1 and FEV1/FVC are low in obstructive disorders such as asthma or chronic obstructive pulmonary disease. The FVC and FEV1 are expressed in liters and in percent predicted of a healthy individual of the same sex, age, and height. It is helpful for your doctors to know these numbers and also to know what the rate of change over time has been.

Children as young as 5 or 6 can cooperate with spirometry. You or your child will likely have spirometry every year to monitor pulmonary function. You will likely have other pulmonary function tests too, such as peak cough flow, which measures the force of your cough (see Question 35).

Forced vital capacity (FVC)

A measure of how much air you can exhale at full capacity, which helps determine the strength of the diaphragm and other respiratory muscles.

Forced expiratory volume measured over 1 second (FEV1)

A measure of how much air can be expelled in the first second of exhalation.

35. What is cough assist?

Cough assist is a technique used when your cough is weak from disease involvement of respiratory muscles. The technique is usually recommended when the FVC (see Question 34) is below 50% of predicted or the peak cough flow is less than 270 liters per minute (L/min). Through use of a machine that is connected to the patient with a mask or a mouthpiece, the cough assist (or insufflator/exsufflator) rapidly shifts from a positive pressure (pushing air in) to a negative pressure (sucking air out), thus simulating a cough.

Cough assist has a number of benefits. The large positive pressure breath prevents the collapse of lung tissue, called **atelectasis**, which can allow infections to take hold. It also stretches the respiratory muscles with benefits similar to stretching of the limbs. The strong negative pressure phase helps expel mucous, sputum, and foreign matter, including bacteria, from the lungs.

Atelectasis
Collapse of lung tissue.

Cough assist should be used at least twice daily, once in the morning and once in the evening, and more frequently when there is an upper respiratory infection or any phlegm buildup. A pulmonologist or respiratory technician will make recommendations for settings, but reasonable initial settings for routine use (no significant phlegm or infection) are +30 inspiratory pressure and −10 expiratory pressure. During periods of increased mucus, sputum, or a respiratory infection, the expiratory pressure should be made more negative (−30 to −40) to simulate a stronger cough.

There are several brands of cough assist machines. Many today are small and simple to use.

Tayjus' Comment:

I cannot speak highly enough about the cough assist. I never used to use it until I got pneumonia. I learned my lesson and realized how useful the cough assist was. I use the cough assist every day when I wake up and sometimes before bed. It always feels good to use for expanding my lungs and clearing phlegm. Now when I have a cold, I use it as often as needed, sometimes using it 7 or 8 times a day. It makes such a difference when I have a cold, and I swear by it. It has gotten me through so many colds. Everyone with DMD really needs to have a cough assist.

36. When should I start using nighttime ventilatory support?

For those whose MD affects the muscles of respiration, problems typically begin at nighttime. In the daytime when we are awake and upright, our respiratory control centers are more active, plus gravity helps pull the diaphragm muscle down and expand the lungs. When you lie down to sleep, breathing is more inefficient, and gravity is no longer helping the diaphragm; therefore, it is harder to breathe.

Common symptoms suggesting that you need help breathing at night include daytime somnolence (feeling sleepy or falling asleep during the day), increased fatigue, difficulty concentrating, morning or continuous headaches, frequent nighttime arousals, nightmares, or awakening with shortness of breath or fast heartbeat. Sometimes, however, the individual with MD will have few or no symptoms of disordered nighttime breathing. Testing is therefore very helpful.

There are two tests that help predict when one needs nighttime ventilatory support. The first is spirometry (see Question 34), which measures pulmonary function. Spirometry allows measurement of the forced vital capacity, or FVC, which is the total amount of air you can exhale starting at full lung capacity. When the FVC becomes less than 50% of what is predicted for a typical person of the same height, age, and sex, then it may signify significant respiratory muscle weakness, and frequently, it means that nighttime ventilator support is needed.

The other test is the polysomnogram or **sleep study**. In a sleep study, electrodes are placed on your head, chest, and limbs to record activity from your brain (to determine if you are sleeping), lungs, heart, and muscles. A sensor on the finger or ear measures the oxygenation level in your blood. There may also be a carbon dioxide sensor. The sleep study will diagnose sleep-disordered breathing such as periods of **apnea** (no breathing), hypoxia (low oxygen), or hypercapnia (high carbon dioxide). A physician specially trained in sleep medicine will make the recommendation for CPAP or BIPAP (see Question 37). Once the need for nighttime ventilator support is determined, the first trial is typically done in the sleep study lab so the correct pressures needed for good oxygenation and sleep are determined in a process called "titration." A respiratory therapist will then be scheduled to come to your house to set up the machine for use.

People who need nighttime ventilatory support are usually ultimately very happy with their support because it gives them a good night's sleep, decreases daytime sleepiness, decreases morning headaches, and increases energy levels.

Sleep study

A study that determines whether nighttime breathing during sleep is adequate using sensors to measure blood oxygen levels, breathing patterns, and brain, heart, and lung activity.

Apnea

The temporary cessation of breathing.

Tayjus' Comment:

I was initially very stubborn when it came to using the BI-PAP. I never felt sleepy or sluggish during the day, and I never had headaches. I also always hated wearing the mask and the sound of the BIPAP. About 5 years ago, I got pneumonia, and that was when I started using the BIPAP. While it is hard to get used to, you do eventually get used to it, and I know I cannot sleep well when I don't use it.

37. What's the difference between BIPAP and CPAP?

BIPAP and CPAP are both forms of noninvasive ventilatory support. BIPAP stands for bilevel positive airway pressure and has two settings of pressure: an inspiratory pressure and an expiratory pressure. CPAP stands for continuous positive airway pressure and has only one pressure setting. BIPAP and CPAP are both provided by small machines the size of a lunch box that provide pressure through a tube to a mask that fits over the nose or nose and mouth.

Obstructive sleep apnea

Interruption of breathing during sleep due to airway obstruction.

CPAP is commonly prescribed for those who have **obstructive sleep apnea,** or interrupted breathing while sleeping. The person inspires on their own and the applied pressure helps keep the airways open during breathing. However, the continuous positive pressure may be difficult to exhale against. BIPAP is used for those with respiratory muscle weakness because it assists with inspiration by generating a higher positive pressure during inspiration. BIPAP can be adjusted to have a lower expiratory pressure to reduce the work of exhaling. BIPAP can also be used for those with sleep apnea and may be more appropriate for patients with sleep apnea and respiratory muscle weakness. BIPAP has an additional feature in that it can set a backup rate of breaths per minute so that a breath is triggered if it is not spontaneously taken. This feature may help people who under-breathe at night. Both BIPAP and CPAP can provide humidified air to reduce dryness in the mouth and lungs.

BIPAP is generally started at nighttime after a sleep study indicates low oxygenation or high carbon dioxide levels (see Question 36). Sometimes, BIPAP is also used during the day if there is respiratory insufficiency or severe respiratory muscle weakness. CPAP is only a support for breathing while sleeping.

Individuals frequently have difficulty adjusting to BIPAP or CPAP initially. The masks can be uncomfortable, and the pressurized air takes getting used to. There are many different types and sizes of masks for different face shapes and sizes. You should experiment with different masks until you find one that you can comfortably sleep in. Some models allow you to gradually increase the pressure so that you can get comfortable with the pressure as you are falling asleep.

Colin's Comment:

I had a love–hate relationship with my CPAP for a long time. I loved the benefits of a restful night's sleep and the lack of grogginess in the morning due to hypoxia. On the other hand, I hated trying to sleep with the mask on, trying to keep the seal, and regulating my sleep patterns. This led to me only using my CPAP for part of the night or not at all. There were periods where I wouldn't use it for months at a time. Using my CPAP can still be a struggle at times, but I think that the combination of my lack of maturity when

I first started using it and my denial that anything was wrong with me is no longer getting in my way. Using my CPAP religiously and continuously and experiencing the benefits night after night took a long time for me to accomplish, and I do still miss a night now and then. However, the combination of sleep apnea and the severe fatigue from MD make it crucial that I use my CPAP to get restful sleep so I can participate in the activities I love and stay healthy.

38. What are the advantages and disadvantages of noninvasive mechanical ventilation?

When respiratory muscle weakness progresses, it may be detected by a fall in FVC and lower oxygen or higher carbon dioxide during sleep. In these cases, it may be necessary to provide breathing support during the night and sometimes during the day. Nighttime noninvasive mechanical ventilation is typically required when the FVC is <50% predicted, or oxygen saturations are consistently less than 89%, or carbon dioxide levels are higher than 50 mm Hg. Significant difficulty breathing while awake and upright, consistent reduction in oxygen saturation, or elevation of CO_2 are often reasons for using noninvasive mechanical ventilation during the day.

Noninvasive mechanical ventilation involves the use of a pressure-cycled ventilator (such as BIPAP) or a volume-cycled ventilator and an "interface" (such as a face mask, nasal pillows, or mouthpiece). See Question 39 for more about mouthpieces and sip and puff ventilation.

With good daytime ventilation, somnolence, fatigue, headaches, and shortness of breath are significantly improved. Other advantages to noninvasive mechanical ventilation include that it preserves the natural nose and mouth barriers to infection and for many feels more natural than the alternative of invasive mechanical ventilation (Question 40).

There are disadvantages also to noninvasive mechanical ventilation. This includes filling of the stomach with air, eye irritation, skin breakdown from some types of interfaces, sinus pain or congestion, and leakage of the mask causing less pressure to be delivered. Sometimes, patients are not able to tolerate the mask interface, or the noninvasive ventilator is not able to correct their breathing abnormalities. Your doctors will work with you to determine what method of ventilation is best for you.

39. What is a sip and puff ventilator?

Sip and puff ventilation is one form of mouthpiece noninvasive ventilation. Mouthpiece ventilation utilizes a variety of oral interfaces that may connect with the ventilator (see Figure 7). It can be used with any form of pressure-cycled ventilator (e.g., BIPAP) or, more commonly, with a volume-cycled ventilator. In sip and puff, the mouthpiece is a straw or tube that is held or suspended so that it is easily accessible to the patient's mouth. The ventilator can be portable, and the whole apparatus can fit on a wheelchair. From the mouthpiece, the individual activates a breath by putting the mouth on the mouthpiece and exerting a small negative pressure, like taking a sip. Exhalation is initiated with a puff.

Mouthpiece ventilation interfaces, including sip and puff mouthpieces, take the place of a face mask, nose mask, or nasal pillows. They therefore have the advantage

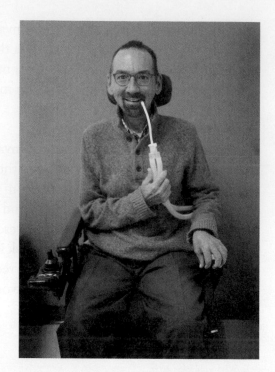

Figure 7 An individual with LGMD holding the mouthpiece to a sip and puff ventilator. Mouthpieces can also be suspended from the wheelchair with gooseneck tubing for those who have arm weakness or want their hands free.

of ease of speaking and swallowing and lack of abrasion to the nose bridge, forehead, or face. Mouthpieces have disadvantages too—they can only be used while awake and require some neck and lip strength to use effectively. Like other noninvasive ventilatory support, they may cause distention of the stomach with air.

40. What are the advantages and disadvantages of invasive mechanical ventilation?

Sometimes respiratory support cannot be managed by noninvasive mechanical ventilation, or secretions cannot be managed with cough assist. In these situations, or because of individual preference, a person with MD may undergo an elective **tracheostomy**, in which a small hole is made in the trachea below the vocal cords and a tube is inserted into the trachea, which then connects to a ventilator. More often than not, tracheostomy follows an acute illness such as a pneumonia in which a hospitalized patient has a breathing tube inserted through his or her mouth to help with respiratory support. Although more hospitals are becoming proficient in transitioning an intubated patient to noninvasive ventilator support after the acute illness, this is sometimes not feasible, and a tracheostomy is offered.

Tracheostomy
Insertion of a tube into the trachea via surgery to connect the trachea to a ventilator and help a patient breathe.

There are some advantages of invasive mechanical ventilation over noninvasive mechanical ventilation. Tracheostomy is indicated if the throat muscles are too weak to protect against having saliva or food going down the trachea into the lungs and causing aspiration pneumonia. Ventilation through a tracheostomy can deliver higher pressures than noninvasive mechanical ventilation, which in some situations may be indicated. Tracheostomy can provide access for direct suctioning of secretions. And there is nothing on the face to interfere with communication or to cause skin breakdown.

There are also disadvantages to invasive mechanical ventilation. The tracheostomy may generate more secretions, which may require frequent suctioning. The risk of infections, such as tracheitis and pneumonia, is higher. The tracheostomy site needs nursing care and cleaning, and the endotracheal tube needs to be changed by a physician periodically. In some states, only nurses can perform tracheostomy and ventilator care, and Medicare may not cover this care in the community.

Contrary to common perception, tracheostomy does not generally worsen swallowing and does not take away the ability to speak. Usually, an individual with a tracheostomy can continue to communicate with a normal voice using a speaking valve.

Whether to pursue noninvasive or invasive mechanical ventilation is often as much as a personal choice as a medical choice. Your pulmonologist, neurologist, and respiratory therapist can help you with this important decision.

41. What are some things to remember when going to the emergency department?

Many things bring people to an emergency department (ED). If you do need to go to an ED, it is important to inform ED staff of your special medical needs. Bear in mind, though, that physicians and staff in the ED are not going to be as familiar with the specific characteristics of diseases like MD as specialists would be, so you should be ready to call their attention to aspects they may overlook.

What does this mean? As an example, it is important to remember to tell them, "No oxygenation without ventilation," particularly if you have respiratory muscle weakness. This is because if you have respiratory muscle weakness and typically use some ventilatory assistance such as a BIPAP, you should not be given supplemental oxygen without ventilatory support. The reason is that you likely retain higher levels of CO_2 than most people, and your respiratory drive is based on the levels of O_2 in your blood. When these O_2 levels become high, as when supplemental oxygen is given, your respiratory drive decreases, your CO_2 increases, and you are at risk of respiratory crisis and altered mentation, including coma. If you need oxygen, for example in the setting of pneumonia, this must be given with ventilatory support. Bring your home BIPAP and cough assist device with you to the ED.

A rare cause of difficulty breathing and change in thinking is **fat embolism syndrome**. This occurs when fat from the bone marrow, such as after a long bone fracture, makes its way to the lungs and causes decreased oxygenation to the brain, body, and other organs. This may not be one of the first things that the ED physicians think of, so it is important to mention this possibility in the setting of bone fracture.

Fat embolism syndrome

A dangerous situation in people who've broken a bone where fat from the bone marrow migrates to the lungs and brain.

If you are on daily steroids at home, then you should receive a higher dose of steroids, called "stress-dose" steroids, in the setting of acute and serious illness. You should give a list of your medications to the ED physicians so this is clear.

For those with DM, painful abdominal distention in what is called a **pseudo-obstruction** can be mistaken for an acute obstruction, appendicitis, or cholangitis. Treatment for a pseudo-obstruction is conservative management with intravenous fluids and medications, while other complications often require surgery. Ask the ED physicians if they have considered this possibility.

Pseudo-obstruction

An abnormality in the coordinated contraction of the intestines that might be mistaken for bowel obstruction.

If surgery and anesthesia are needed, many individuals with MD should avoid inhaled anesthesia, although IV anesthesia is considered safe. One muscle relaxant used in conjunction with anesthesia, succinylcholine, should always be avoided (see Question 72). For some MDs such as DM, recovery from anesthesia may take longer and additional monitoring should be performed.

As discussed earlier in Question 2, the enzymes aspartate aminotransferase (AST) and alanine aminotransferase (AST) are released into the blood by muscle and liver. Measurements of these enzymes in the blood are frequently called "liver function tests," and many physicians will see elevated levels and think you have a liver injury. However, AST and ALT are frequently elevated at baseline in patients with MD due to their muscle disease. If there is other concern for a liver injury (such as in the case of a toxic ingestion), then the gamma glutamyl transferase (GGT) test is a more specific marker of liver function that can be used instead.

The major reservoir of potassium in the body is muscle. In people with MD, muscle mass can be quite low. It is therefore important that when potassium is given to people with advanced MD, it must be given slowly and checked frequently. It is easy to overshoot potassium repletion in the setting of low muscle mass.

In summary, many ED physicians may not be familiar with MD and all of these related concepts. It is good to carry a card with you on appropriate emergency management such as "No oxygenation without ventilation," particularly if you have respiratory muscle weakness. Bringing baseline test results such as your electrocardiogram (see Question 42), echocardiogram, and pulmonary function tests can be very helpful. Have the telephone numbers of your neurologist, cardiologist, and pulmonologist to give to the ED physicians so that they can call to better understand your condition and discuss your care.

PART SIX

The Heart

Why do I need an electrocardiogram?

What is an echocardiogram?

How can I protect my heart?

More . . .

42. Why do I need an electrocardiogram?

MD may involve not only the muscles of your face and limbs but also the muscles of your internal organs. Many MDs involve cardiac muscle and are associated with disturbance of the electrical activity of the heart (leading to abnormal or irregular heart rhythms called **cardiac arrhythmias**) or impairment of the heart's pumping function (leading to cardiomyopathy). Therefore, it is important for many individuals with MD to have a heart specialist (cardiologist) as part of his or her medical team. MDs associated with cardiac disorders include DMD, DM, BMD, EDMD, and some, but not all, of the LGMDs, DDs, and CMDs. An **electrocardiogram** (**ECG**, or sometimes **EKG**) is one way in which your cardiologist will assess the health of your heart and should be done for those at risk at least once a year.

The pump function of the heart is coordinated by electrical activity. An electrical impulse travels through the heart and makes the heart beat in a synchronized manner. Any disruptions to this regular electrical activity may result in abnormal heart rhythms (arrhythmias) and lead to a number of problems, such as palpitations, fainting, or even sudden death.

Arrhythmias may make your heart unable to pump as much blood as needed. An ECG is one way to quickly measure this electrical impulse traveling through the heart. It is obtained by connecting small electrode patches to the skin of your chest, arms, and legs. It takes a few minutes to connect the electrodes and a few seconds to get a recording. An ECG does not hurt. By measuring how long the electrical wave takes

Cardiac arrhythmia

An irregular or abnormal heartbeat rhythm.

Electrocardiogram (ECG, EKG)

A test that records the electrical signals in your heart. It's a common test used to detect heart problems and monitor the heart's status in many situations.

to travel from one part of the heart to the next, it informs the cardiologist on whether the electrical activity is normal, slow, or fast and whether it is regular or irregular.

Of note, an ECG provides only a brief (10-second) recording of the electrical activity of your heart. If your cardiologist suspects that you have an arrhythmia, but no abnormalities are captured on the routine ECG, you may be asked to wear a Holter monitor, which provides a more representative snapshot of your heart's electrical activity. The Holter is a portable ECG that checks the electrical activity of your heart for 24 or 48 hours. Additionally, there are portable ECGs, called event monitors, that can measure your ECG for up to 30 days if your symptoms are so infrequent that they are unlikely be captured on a 24-hour recording (e.g., symptoms that occur only once a week or every other week). You will wear a battery-operated recording device around your neck or waist and are asked not to get the device wet. You will also be asked to keep a diary of any symptoms that you have such as palpitations while you are wearing the Holter or event monitor.

If you have rhythm abnormalities that happen infrequently, your cardiologist may recommend an implantable loop recorder. An implantable loop recorder is about the size of a small USB stick that is inserted under the skin in the chest using local anesthesia and can record the heartbeat continuously for up to three years.

43. What is an echocardiogram?

An echocardiogram is a safe, noninvasive way to evaluate the pump function of the heart. High-frequency sound waves (ultrasound, which does not involve radiation) are used to create pictures of the heart. From these pictures, the cardiologist can determine the size and strength of the various chambers in your heart, evaluate the structure and function of your heart valves, and look for any abnormalities, such as a blood clot in the heart.

During an echocardiogram, you will be asked to undress from the waist up. ECG electrodes will be attached to your chest and limbs. Gel will be applied to a probe, which then will be pressed against your chest. The test may last up to 30 minutes, and it is painless, although the gel can initially be cold! For some individuals (particularly in the setting of chest deformities), it is hard to get good pictures of the heart through an echo-cardiogram, and a cardiac MRI may be ordered instead. Cardiac MRI is also a noninvasive and safe procedure.

With every heartbeat, blood is pumped from the two main chambers (ventricles) in the heart. During the relaxation phase (diastole), the ventricle fills with blood, and during the contraction phase (systole), the ventricle pumps out the blood. Not all the blood that enters the ventricle is pumped out. The percentage of blood that is pumped out is called the **ejection fraction**. The left ventricular ejection fraction is a good measure of the strength of the heart and can be estimated by an echocardiogram or a cardiac MRI (see **Figure 8**). A normal ejection fraction is greater than 55%. If you have an MD that is associated with cardiomyopathy (disease of the heart muscle) then your cardiologist will follow your ejection fraction and other parameters through echocardiograms, usually on a yearly basis.

Ejection fraction

The percent of blood volume that the ventricles send out to the body. The ejection fraction is an important measure of cardiac function.

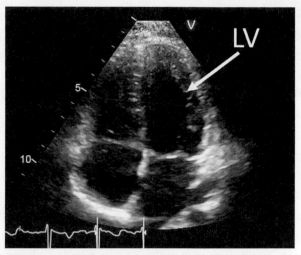

Figure 8 An echocardiogram of a DMD boy showing all four chambers of the heart, including the left ventricle (LV) that pumps blood to the body.

Image courtesy of W. Reid Thompson.

44. How can I protect my heart?

Everyone should take preventative steps to protect their heart. This is particularly important, however, for those who have an MD that affects the heart. Individuals with some MDs are at risk of cardiomyopathy (weakening of the heart muscles) and cardiac arrhythmias (abnormal rhythms of the heart). All individuals can also have more common forms of cardiovascular disease related to aging, such as disease of the blood vessels supplying the heart muscle (also known as coronary artery disease), just like the general population.

One of the key aspects to good heart health is blood pressure. High blood pressure increases the work of the heart, and management of blood pressure is one of the key measures that one can take to prevent the onset or worsening of cardiomyopathy. High blood pressure also increases cardiovascular disease and the risk of heart attack. Your cardiologist may recommend that you take medications to decrease the work of the heart. There are also lifestyle interventions that you can make to lower your blood pressure such as getting regular aerobic exercise (see Question 17), limiting your salt intake, losing excess weight (see Question 49), and reducing alcohol consumption.

Elevated cholesterol leads to cardiovascular disease and increased risk of heart attack. A diet rich in fruits and vegetables and low in saturated fats and cholesterol along with regular exercise are important interventions to reduce cholesterol. A nutritionist can help you evaluate your diet and make recommended changes. If these interventions are not enough to keep cholesterol in a healthy range, then your doctor may prescribe a cholesterol-lowering drug. Some of these drugs, such as statins, have known muscle side effects. Although individuals with MD are not more prone to muscle side effects from statins, it may be hard to differentiate the side effect from statins from the progression of MD. To avoid any additional insult to the muscles, alternatives to statin therapy are suggested, if possible.

Individuals with DM are at higher than average risk of prediabetes and type 2 diabetes. Both prediabetes and diabetes are linked to cardiovascular disease and heart attacks. The hemoglobin A1C and glucose tolerance tests are blood tests that can be performed by your doctor to determine whether you have diabetes or prediabetes. If you do, your doctor may recommend a nutritional evaluation, an exercise regimen, and potentially medications.

Tobacco use is the greatest risk factor for developing cardiovascular disease. It is crucial that you not smoke cigarettes or other tobacco products. There are nicotine replacement therapies and prescription medications available to help you stop smoking. You can call 1-800-QUIT-NOW for additional assistance.

Finally, exercise, in addition to lowering blood pressure and reducing insulin resistance, has direct benefits to heart muscle. But it can be difficult to exercise when you have MD. You may be able to set up a walking program or use a stationary bike. Or if you are nonambulatory, you may be able to participate in aquatic therapy. It may take some creativity along with the help of your doctors to figure out how to best stay active.

45. What is a pacemaker?

A pacemaker is a small battery-operated device that is used in the setting of a heart rhythm that is too slow. Tests that indicate that you might need a pacemaker include ECG or Holter monitor (see Question 42), echocardiogram (see Question 43), or an **electrophysiology study**. An electrophysiology study is a test of the heart's electrical system in which a wire is inserted through a vein to the heart and electrically stimulates your heart to see how your heart's electrical system responds. These tests may pick up arrhythmias for which a **pacemaker** could be helpful, including slower-than-normal heartbeats or long pauses between heartbeats. Without a pacemaker, these arrhythmias result in not enough blood being pumped to the brain and body and may make you feel faint, fatigued, or even lose consciousness.

A pacemaker consists of a battery-operated generator and leads. The battery-operated generator is usually placed under the skin below your collar bone. It is a small metal container about the size of a matchbox that

Electrophysiology study

A test of the heart's electrical system in which a wire is inserted through a vein to the heart and electrically stimulates your heart to see how your heart's electrical system responds.

Pacemaker

A battery-operated device implanted under the skin that monitors the heart's electrical activity and supplies electrical impulses when an irregularity occurs.

monitors and regulates the electrical activity of your heart. The generator is connected to your heart with one to three insulated wires (called leads) and continuously records the electrical activity of your heart. If your heart rate is normal, it only monitors your heart activity. In case of a slow heartbeat, however, it can generate electrical impulses to stimulate or "pace" your heart. You do not feel these electrical signals.

Pacemaker insertion is a minor surgery, after which you will be asked to stay in the hospital overnight. Pacemaker insertion usually does not require general anesthesia. The pacemaker battery lasts for 8–12 years (depending, among other things, on how much pacing you need). When the pacemaker battery is running low, your cardiologist will change the pacemaker generator, but usually not the leads. Changing the pacemaker generator is an outpatient procedure.

There are three main types of pacemakers:

1. A *single-chamber pacemaker* carries electrical impulses to the right ventricle (the lower right chamber of your heart, which pumps blood to the lungs). Of note, *single-chamber leadless pacemakers* now exist as well; these are implanted directly in the heart.

2. A *dual-chamber pacemaker* carries electrical impulses to both the right atrium (the upper right chamber of the heart that pumps to the right ventricle) and the right ventricle.

3. A *biventricular pacemaker*, also called *cardiac resynchronization therapy (CRT)*, stimulates both the right ventricle and the left ventricle (the lower left chamber of your heart that pumps blood to the body). This type of pacemaker is

used in those with heart failure and a slowing of electrical activity with the left chamber of the heart called a *left bundle branch block*.

A pacemaker is not to be confused with an *implantable cardioverter-defibrillator (ICD)*. Like pacemakers, ICDs also continuously monitor the electrical activity of your heart, but in contrast to pacemakers, ICDs are primarily designed to treat fast, life-threatening heart rhythm disorders, which pacemakers cannot do (see Question 46).

Essentially, a pacemaker is a little computer with a battery. The pacemaker runs daily self-checks to ensure that its hardware, battery, and leads are working well. Your cardiologist will be able to remotely monitor your pacemaker with a Bluetooth-enabled device that you place next to your bed. During the night, this Bluetooth-enabled remote monitor will establish contact with your pacemaker, and, if one parameter of the pacemaker function is flagged as abnormal, a message will be automatically sent to your cardiologist's office. Remote monitoring is an additional safety feature and has the advantage that you don't need to see your cardiologist in person to check your pacemaker every three months. With remote pacemaker monitoring enabled, usually only one in-person visit per year is necessary to check the pacemaker.

Most household electrical appliances, including microwaves, do *not* interfere with the pacemaker. However, you must take certain precautions if you have a pacemaker. You cannot go near large power-generating equipment such as high-voltage transformers. Most modern pacemakers are MRI-conditional, which means that you can have MRI scans as long as the pacemaker is monitored. Your pacemaker may set off the detection of airport security, and you should not let the security agent hold a handheld scanner over your chest for more than a few seconds, as it may disrupt the pacemaker's function (it is important to warn security personnel that you have this device in advance of screening). If you are scheduled for surgery, you should inform the surgeon that you have a pacemaker. Carrying a wallet card with information on your pacemaker or wearing a medical alert bracelet is helpful.

46. What is an implantable cardioverter defibrillator?

Implantable cardioverter defibrillator (ICD)

An implanted device that continuously monitors heart rhythm and provides high-intensity electrical impulses to restore a normal rhythm if a life-threatening arrhythmia occurs.

An **implantable cardioverter defibrillator (ICD)** is an implanted device used to prevent sudden cardiac death. It monitors your heart rhythm continuously and, in case a fast and life-threatening heart rhythm is detected, it can provide high intensity electrical impulses (defibrillation or electrical shocks) to restore a normal rhythm. This high-intensity shock that an ICD can provide when you have a life-threatening arrhythmia is something a pacemaker does not do. The ICD also records and stores information about your heart rhythm, and any electrical impulses delivered by the ICD, for your cardiologist to review.

You might need an ICD if your heart's lower chambers (the ventricles) are at risk of a dangerously abnormal rhythm that could lead to a cardiac arrest. Your cardiologist might also recommend an ICD if your ejection fraction (the percent of blood volume that the ventricles send out to the body) is below 35%. This degree of cardiomyopathy puts you at risk of life-threatening arrhythmias. Similar to a pacemaker (see Question 45), tests that might indicate you need an ICD include an ECG, Holter or event monitor, echocardiogram, cardiac MRI, or electrophysiology study.

Like the pacemaker, the ICD consists of a generator and leads inserted under the skin below the collarbone. The battery-powered generator is usually twice as large as that of a pacemaker—about the size of a stopwatch—and is connected to insulated wires called leads, which are anchored in the heart and which monitor the heart rhythm and deliver a shock as needed. Implantation of an ICD is a minor surgery that requires an overnight hospitalization. Insertion of an ICD usually does not require general anesthesia. The ICD battery lasts for 6–14 years (depending on, among other reasons, how much pacing you need and how many shocks are delivered by the device). When the ICD battery is running low, your cardiologist will change the ICD generator, but usually not the leads. Changing the generator is an outpatient procedure.

Most ICDs can function as a pacemaker and provide low-intensity electrical impulses that are not felt. Therefore, similar to pacemakers, ICDs exist as single-chamber, dual-chamber, or biventricular (CRT) devices. Importantly, an ICD may have a pacemaker function, but a pacemaker can never function as an ICD, as only ICDs can deliver high-intensity shocks for life-threatening fast arrhythmias. Unlike the small electrical impulses that are delivered by a pacemaker or an ICD with a pacemaker function, the high-intensity electrical impulse from an ICD is very powerful and can feel like a kick to the chest. Appropriate shocks generally occur very infrequently and, although unpleasant and painful, can be lifesaving. In rare instances, the ICD can fire inappropriately, and if that happens, the device needs to be reprogrammed.

Just like a pacemaker, an ICD is a little computer with a battery that runs daily self-checks to ensure that its hardware, battery, and leads are working well. And as with the pacemaker, your cardiologist has the ability to remotely monitor your ICD with a Bluetooth-enabled device that you place next to your bed; this device will notify your cardiologist's office if any abnormalities are seen in your heart function. Again, this remote monitoring is an additional safety feature that means you won't need to see your cardiologist in person to check your ICD every three months but instead will visit once per year to check the ICD, as long as there are no incidents, such as a defibrillation shock, requiring closer review.

The ICD has similar limits in regards to magnetic fields and power-generating equipment to those related to a pacemaker (see Question 45). Most modern ICDs, like pacemakers, are MRI-conditional, which means that you can have MRI scans as long as the ICD is monitored. The same precautions regarding security scanners apply when traveling. You should carry a card or wear a bracelet indicating that you have an ICD.

47. What are advance directives?

Advance directives are legal documents that help you direct your health care if you become unable to communicate your wishes. Advance directives include **living wills** and **durable power of attorney for health care**.

The durable power of attorney for health care identifies another person who has the authority to make medical decisions for you if you are unable. This person is called a *proxy*, *agent*, or *surrogate*. Most people choose a close friend or family member to take on this responsibility. However, it could be a lawyer, clergyman, or doctor. It

Living will

A legal document that describes your preferences for what treatments should be performed or not performed if you be unable to express them.

Durable power of attorney for health care

A legal document that identifies another person who can make medical decisions for you if you cannot.

is important that this person can understand the treatment options, your values, and your preferences.

Your preferences for treatment are explained in a living will. These preferences go into effect only if you are incapacitated and unable to speak for yourself. Some of the decisions about which a healthcare provider would need to know your preferences include when and whether to initiate cardiopulmonary resuscitation, put in an endotracheal tube for mechanical ventilation, provide tube feeding or intravenous fluids, or initiate organ and tissue donation. It is helpful to talk to your doctor about these end-of-life issues before drawing up your advance directives. Most states have their own advance directive forms, and it is helpful to use the state forms where you reside to avoid confusion. One site that provides all state forms is: https://www.aarp.org/caregiving/financial-legal/free-printable-advance-directives/. Some states require that the advance directives be witnessed, and a few require your signature to be notarized. It is not necessary to use a lawyer. Once you have written your living will and durable power of attorney for health care, give copies to your healthcare proxy and to your doctors.

Every adult should have healthcare directives. You can revise your directives at any time, and it is a good idea to revisit them every 10 years or so. You may never face a medical situation where you are unable to speak for yourself and make your wishes known. However, having healthcare directives ensures that you are treated in a way that conforms with your values and preferences.

PART SEVEN

Eating and Nutrition

What are some nutritional recommendations?

What is a healthy weight?

Does alcohol affect muscles?

More . . .

48. What are some nutritional recommendations?

Proper nutrition is important for the health of your muscles as well as your other organs. There is not enough research on whether individuals with MD have unique nutritional needs to make specific recommendations. However, the 2015 U.S. Dietary Guidelines for Americans recommends the following:

- A variety of vegetables from all of the subgroups— dark green, red, and orange, legumes (beans and peas), starchy, and other
- Fruits, especially whole fruits
- Grains, at least half of which are whole grains
- Fat-free or low-fat dairy, including milk, yogurt, cheese, and/or fortified soy beverages
- A variety of protein foods, including seafood, lean meats and poultry, eggs, legumes (beans and peas), and nuts, seeds, and soy products

The total calories that you should take in during a day is dependent on weight, activity level, body composition, age, and gender. This number can be estimated by a nutritionist. It is good to have a consultation with a nutritionist to determine calorie needs, assess if micro- and macronutrient needs are being met, and identify specific nutritional goals. A nutritionist will also teach you how to read nutritional information on food labels, which includes calories per serving. Because corticosteroids can lead to increased appetite and weight gain, every individual with MD should have a nutrition consult before initiating corticosteroids.

Many patients wonder how much protein, fat, and carbohydrates should be consumed daily. This varies significantly between patients, but you should strive for a balanced diet where 45–65% of your calories are from carbohydrates, 20–35% from fat, and 10–35% from protein. It is important that you get adequate protein but taking in excessive protein does not lead to increased muscle size and function. The recommended dietary allowance for protein is 0.95 g/kg body weight per day for children age 4–13 years, 0.85 g/kg per day for children age 14–18 years, and 0.8 g/kg per day for adults age 19 years and older. Again, a nutritionist can identify appropriate daily intake goals for these macronutrients.

Because loss of bone density occurs with corticosteroid use and with immobility, it is crucial to get enough calcium to help maintain strong bones. Dietary sources of calcium are the most easily absorbed, but if you cannot get enough calcium from dietary sources due to food allergies or other reasons, then over-the-counter calcium carbonate or calcium citrate supplements can fill this gap. The recommended daily allowance is 1000 mg for children age 4–8 years, 1300 mg for children age 9–18 years, 1000 mg for adults age 19–50 years, 1000 mg for men age 51–70, 1200 mg for women age 51–70, and 1200 mg for adults age 71 and above. Calculators of calcium intake can be found online to help determine if you are consuming enough. Similarly, a multivitamin can be added to make sure you are getting the proper micronutrients. There is more on vitamin D supplementation in Question 56.

Frequently, individuals with MD do not drink adequate amounts of fluids due to the difficulty with using the bathroom. This can lead to kidney stones and constipation. You should strive for 1.2 liters of liquids per day (approximately 5 cups) for children age 4–8 years, 1.8 liters (approximately 8 cups) for children age 9–13 years, 2.6 liters (approximately 11 cups) for children age 14–18 years, and 3.0 liters (approximately 13 cups) for adults aged 19 years or older. Try to get most of these fluid requirements through water, as other fluids are high in sugar and calories. Caffeinated beverages such as soda, tea, and coffee increase urination and result in loss of fluids, so avoid them.

Individuals with MD are more likely to suffer from constipation due to decreased activity, inadequate fluid consumption (see previous paragraph), medication use, and alterations in body composition. Therefore, it is important for the individual with MD to consume adequate dietary fiber to promote bowel regularity. To obtain the recommended number of grams of dietary fiber a child or teenager should consume daily, take the child's age and add 5—so, for instance, a 10-year-old boy should consume 15 grams fiber daily ($10 + 5 = 15$ grams of fiber). Adults should consume 25–30 grams fiber daily regardless of age. Fortunately, eating a healthy, balanced diet rich in whole grains, fruits, and vegetables ensures adequate dietary fiber consumption.

While you want to aim to maintain a healthy weight (see Question 49), you should eat when you are hungry and not skip meals. When fasting, the body utilizes muscle and fat stores as a source of energy and to maintain blood glucose levels. Don't skip breakfast!

Finally, when setting dietary goals for the individual with MD, it is helpful to have the whole family participate in healthy eating. Work with your nutritionist to plan out healthy, balanced meals that can benefit the whole family.

49. What is a healthy weight?

For optimum health and function it is helpful to have an average weight. If you are underweight, you risk not having enough nutrients for optimal muscle health.

During periods of fasting such as overnight and stress such as illness, you need enough fat stores in order that the body will not use muscle stores to maintain blood glucose levels. It is good to have just a little excess weight in reserve for these times.

On the other hand, being overweight has significant health risks. Being overweight increases the risk of diabetes, high blood pressure, and high blood cholesterol with associated cardiovascular risks (Question 44). It is also harder to move a large body than a smaller body, and as muscle strength declines, weight can play a substantial role in motor function.

The body mass index (BMI) is a good indicator of healthy weight for most people. The BMI is the weight in kilograms divided by the square of height in meters. A healthy BMI for adults is between 18.5 kg/m^2 and 24.9 kg/m^2. Less than 18.5 kg/m^2 is underweight and between 25 kg/m^2 and 29.9 kg/m^2 is overweight. A BMI over 30 kg/m^2 is considered obese. For children, it is important to take into account the age and gender of the individual. This gives you a BMI-for-age percentile specific for girls or boys. The goal is to have a weight between the 10th and 85th percentiles on standard growth charts. If the height cannot be measured because the individual is nonambulatory and/ or has severe contractures, height can be estimated from a calculation using the length of the ulna bone (from the elbow to wrist). Since patients with MD have altered body composition, the use of standard growth charts is not ideal. Nevertheless, BMI is easy to obtain, and an experienced professional should be available to interpret the results when working with patients with MD. The Centers for Disease Control and Prevention has a website to calculate your BMI for children and adults: https://www.cdc.gov/healthy weight/assessing/bmi/index.html.

50. Does alcohol affect muscles?

Alcohol adversely affects muscle mass and function. It does this by impacting pathways of muscle mass maintenance and by increasing inflammation and oxidative stress.

Binge drinking, characterized by the consumption of multiple alcoholic drinks during a single episode, resulting in a blood alcohol level of 0.08 g/dL or above, causes breakdown of muscle tissue and elevations in the muscle enzyme, creatine kinase, in the blood and muscle pigment, myoglobin, in the urine. This acute alcoholic **myopathy** (muscle disorder) is frequently characterized by weakness, tenderness, and swelling of affected muscles. The breakdown of muscle from binge drinking can be harmful to kidneys and in severe cases lead to kidney failure. Recovery of muscle in healthy individuals is within days to weeks.

Myopathy

Disorder of muscle.

Lower levels of chronic alcohol consumption can also adversely affect muscles. With continued alcohol use, there is a gradual progression of painless loss of muscle mass and strength. This is a more common form of alcoholic myopathy than acute alcoholic myopathy. It may take several weeks to months to recover from chronic alcoholic myopathy.

It is important to note that none of the studies of alcohol and myopathy was done in patients with MD. It is not known whether patients with MD may be more susceptible to damage from alcohol or, more likely, take longer to regenerate from the harmful effects of alcohol.

It is not known what a safe dose of alcohol is for those with MD, but an occasional glass of wine or beer is unlikely to cause harm.

51. What's involved in a swallowing study?

Sometimes the muscles associated with swallowing are affected in MD. This is particularly true of OPMD, DM, and DMD but can be true of other MDs as well. When you swallow, food normally passes from the mouth to the back of your throat, called the pharynx, and into the esophagus, which leads to the stomach. Contraction of a series of muscles makes the food move in the right direction. In **dysphagia**, these muscles don't work properly. When you have dysphagia, you are much more likely to have small amounts of food or liquid enter your lungs. This is called **aspiration**. You may notice aspiration by a need to cough during or right after eating. You may develop aspiration pneumonia, a lung infection. Other symptoms of dysphagia are a feeling that food gets stuck in your esophagus, difficulty coordinating breathing and swallowing, the need for additional time to swallow, and unexplained weight loss. These and other symptoms would prompt your doctor to order a **swallowing study**.

A swallowing study uses X-rays to film you as you swallow. You will be asked to swallow a chalky drink the consistency of a milk shake with barium sulfate, which is a metallic compound that can be visualized by X-ray. You may also be asked to swallow a solid such as a barium-coated cookie. You will be asked to swallow barium at various different angles. The barium coats the lining of and fills the esophagus. A radiologist will

Dysphagia
Difficulty swallowing.

Aspiration
Having saliva or food enter the trachea instead of the esophagus. This can lead to choking or pneumonia.

Swallowing study
Using X-rays to watch what happens in your mouth, throat, and esophagus as you swallow a special compound visible to the X-ray.

watch the path the barium takes through your upper digestive system as you swallow, either as a movie or still pictures. The procedure generally takes about 30 minutes. The swallowing study may reveal problems in the mouth, pharynx, esophagus, or stomach.

A swallowing study is generally a very safe procedure. The amount of exposure to radiation is small, and you will wear a lead apron to minimize exposure; however, you should not undergo this test if you are pregnant. There are some risks including the possibility that you have an allergic reaction to the barium or that you aspirate some of the barium. You may be constipated from the barium after the procedure. You should drink lots of water following the procedure to minimize constipation.

With the results of a swallowing study, your doctor will be able to assess your ability to swallow safely. He or she may make recommendations for diet modifications, speech and swallowing rehabilitation, or in some cases a gastrostomy tube (see Question 52).

52. What is a gastrostomy tube?

If a swallowing study indicates significant dysphagia or aspiration, if you are suffering recurrent aspiration pneumonias, or if you are unable to eat enough calories by mouth to maintain your weight, a gastrostomy tube or G-tube may be recommended.

A G-tube is a feeding tube that lies on the outside of your abdomen and is directly connected through the skin to your stomach. The feeding tube may sound scary, but it requires a relatively simple procedure to insert and only a small amount of day-to-day care. If there is no increased risk of aspiration, the individual may still want to eat by mouth for pleasure but use the gastrostomy tube for the ease of getting full nutrition and hydration. In addition to nutritional support, gastrostomy tubes can be used to deliver medications, decompress a stomach that is full of air, and reduce the likelihood of aspiration. Most liquid medications can be taken by the G-tube, but for solid pills, individuals should check with the pharmacist or healthcare provider to see if they can be crushed first.

G-tubes can be placed endoscopically, surgically, or radiologically. In an endoscopic approach, a flexible tube (the endoscope) with a light and camera attached to it is slipped down the esophagus into the stomach. The light from the endoscope shines through the skin allowing the surgeon to make a hole (or stoma) in the area over the stomach. This is called a percutaneous endoscopic gastrostomy (PEG) and is frequently the procedure of choice. If there have been prior abdominal surgeries, or if there is an esophageal obstruction or a bleeding disorder, then a surgical approach is usually performed in which a small incision is made in the abdomen. Finally, a G-tube can be inserted using X-ray guidance. You may require general anesthesia or sedation for the procedure. You may go home after being observed for a couple hours or remain in the hospital for 1 or 2 days depending on what type of procedure you had.

The G-tube will be secured in your abdomen and stomach by an internal water-filled balloon or a disc. You will initially have a tube that is up to a foot in length with a one-way valve on the end, often called a PEG tube. However, this long tube can be replaced after the stoma heals with a low-profile button (Figure 9). The button looks like the valve used to inflate a beachball. A button requires an extension tube be used for feedings but has the advantage of lying flat against the stomach and being easily hidden under clothing.

A G-tube requires a little care. The area around the G-tube should be cleaned with soap and water daily. Most tubes do not require a dressing, but sometimes a gauze pad is helpful to catch small amounts of drainage. You should rotate the tube with each feeding. If you have a PEG tube, then you will need to tape the tube to the outside of your abdomen or wear an abdominal binder that holds the tube in place. The tube needs to be replaced every few months which, for a button, can be done at home. You should flush the tube with 10–15 mL of warm water after every feeding or medication to prevent clogging. Sometimes the tube gets dislodged, and then it is important to get a new tube in quickly, as the stoma can close up, requiring another procedure.

A nutritionist will help you determine the best composition and quantity of tube feeds. Feedings can be delivered by one of a few different methods. The tube feed can be delivered with a syringe in a bolus a few times a day. Alternatively, a bag of liquid food can be allowed to drip into the tube by gravity over several minutes to an hour. Finally, a pump can deliver the feed continuously over several hours. This can conveniently be done overnight while you sleep.

G-tubes are not as scary as they sound. They can increase the quality of life by providing proper nutrition when the work of eating has become too burdensome, leading to enhanced health and energy. They can also increase life span through proper nutrition and decreased risk of aspiration.

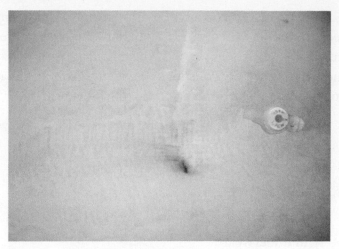

Figure 9 Low profile G-tube button.

53. Is constipation a symptom of muscular dystrophy?

Gastrointestinal (GI) symptoms, including constipation, are common in MDs. Many of the MDs affect the smooth muscle that lines the digestive tract in addition to skeletal muscles, which move the trunk and limbs. However, the causes of constipation are often multifactorial and more complex than just poor muscle activity. Dietary habits and decreased physical activity are common factors contributing to constipation in MDs. Medications such as opioids can contribute to constipation. Various behavioral factors also cause constipation, and these are often overlooked. Studies have shown that children with chronic constipation often have unrecognized behavioral and developmental issues, such as anxiety, attention deficit, hyperactivity, oppositional behaviors, obsessive–compulsive behaviors, or autism.

Constipation in MD is underdiagnosed and undertreated. Most people believe that constipation means reduced frequency or inability to pass stool. What many people, including many medical practitioners, do not realize is that a person can pass one or more stools a day and still be severely constipated. Diagnosis of constipation can be made from any of the following criteria:

1. Not having a bowel movement for 4 or more days
2. Passing very firm or hard stool
3. Having to strain to pass stool
4. Having very large stools
5. Having stool accidents or small smears of stool in underwear

Once diagnosed or suspected, constipation in those with MD should be evaluated and supervised by a medical provider. Prolonged constipation or undertreated constipation can lead to discomfort, hemorrhoids, small cracks or fissures in the anus, fecal impactions, or respiratory compromise.

The recommendations for treating constipation will depend on the severity of the constipation. Those with mild constipation could be treated with increasing water and fiber intake. If not able to increase fiber-containing foods due to picky eating, a fiber supplement could be added to the diet, such as fiber wafers or cookies, fiber gummies, or adding fiber powders to food and drinks.

Medical therapies should be started for moderate to severe constipation. The first line of medical therapy is typically a stool softener, such as polyethylene glycol, lactulose, docusate sodium, and magnesium hydroxide. Stool softeners do not stimulate a person to have a bowel movement, they just hold water into the stool and make it softer. The goal should be to make the stools very soft, so it is easy to pass the stools.

Sometimes a stimulant is used to help improve the ability of the colon to push stool out or increase the frequency of bowel movements. There are primarily two types of stimulant laxatives: senna and bisacodyl. Unlike the stool softeners, these two medications stimulate the need to have a bowel movement. The time of day when stimulants are given needs to be considered in those with MD who are not able to get to a bathroom easily on their own. Your healthcare provider may recommend that these medications are taken in middle of the afternoon or at bedtime with goal of stimulating a bowel movement during the evening or the early morning, when the person with MD has others around to help him or her get to bathroom so that toileting will not interfere with daily activities.

PART EIGHT

Bone Health

What is a DEXA scan?

How can I improve bone density?

How much vitamin D should I take?

More . . .

54. What is a DEXA scan?

Dual-energy X-ray absorptiometry (DEXA)

An imaging method that uses X-ray to assess bone density and body composition.

DEXA (also abbreviated DXA) stands for **dual-energy X-ray absorptiometry**. It measures bone mineral density (BMD) as well as body composition, such as the percent of muscle and fat. The test uses two X-ray beams to take images of soft tissue and bone. DEXA scans can assess either limited parts of your body, such as the lower spine and hips, or the whole body. The noninvasive test is painless and takes 10 to 30 minutes to complete, during which you will be asked to lie on a padded table. The amount of radiation received is less than that of a chest or dental X-ray.

BMD is a measure of the strength or fragility of bones and predicts the likelihood of fracture. Patients with MD may have low BMD for a variety of reasons: Corticosteroids reduce BMD. Decreased weight bearing is also associated with loss of BMD. Finally, weakness of muscles in and of itself may lead to less stress on bones and thus less BMD. For these reasons, a baseline DEXA scan is recommended for most people with MD. Follow-up DEXA scans may be recommended depending on the degree of BMD to monitor progression or to evaluate the effectiveness of prescribed treatments. A DEXA is particularly important if you are falling, have unexplained back pain, or have had a fracture after minimal trauma.

DEXA results are reported in a couple of different ways, either by T-score or Z-score. T-scores and Z-scores represent how many standard deviations an individual is from the average. In regard to BMD, one standard deviation is equal to a 10–12% difference in bone mass.

For adults, a T-score is utilized to interpret the results. The T-score compares your BMD to that of a young adult (20-year-old) of the same gender with peak bone mass. A T-score of 0 would mean that your BMD does not differ from the average 20-year-old. A score of −1 or above is considered normal. A score of −1.1 to −2.4 is considered osteopenic (low bone mass). This means that you have a bone density 10% to 25% below an average healthy young adult. A score of −2.5 or below is considered osteoporotic (porous bone that can lead to fractures). This means that you have a BMD 25% or more below that of an average healthy young adult.

For children, the Z-score is utilized to interpret results. The Z-score compares your BMD to a person of the same age and gender. Z-scores can also be adjusted for pubertal status and height. As children are rapidly growing and gaining bone mass, comparisons to age-matched peers is more useful than comparisons to a healthy adult. For children, a Z-score below −2 is considered low bone mass. The diagnosis of osteoporosis in children is from a combination of fracture history and BMD Z-score.

The DEXA scan provides information about your BMD and risk of fracture. This is important information for any patient with MD, and, as described in Question 55, there are active steps that you can do to increase bone density if a DEXA scan suggests that it is low.

55. How can I improve my bone density?

Good BMD is imperative to prevent fractures, which can be painful and disabling. As described in the previous question, patients with MD are at risk for low BMD for a variety of reasons. Luckily, there are steps you can take to increase low bone density:

- **Nutrition**: Adequate intake of calcium (see Question 48) and vitamin D (see Question 56) is essential for healthy bones. Other important vitamins and minerals for bones can be found in green leafy vegetables and whole grain breads and pastas.

- Exercise: Weight bearing activity improves BMD. Ideally, this would come in the form of aerobic exercise several times a week (see Question 17). However, for those whose weakness is advanced, this may not be possible. In these situations, the use of a stander (see Question 95) to allow weight bearing in a supportive system is helpful.

- Weight: Maintaining a healthy weight is essential for healthy bones. People who are underweight have a higher risk of osteoporosis. People who are overweight put additional stress on bones. You should avoid rapid weight loss and cycling between gaining and losing weight. This may be associated with bone density loss.

- Stop smoking: Smoking increases the risk of osteoporosis and fractures.

- Avoid excessive alcohol and caffeine: Chronic heavy alcohol and/or caffeine consumption is linked to poor calcium absorption and osteoporosis.

- Medications: If you have made the above modifications to your diet and lifestyle and still have osteoporosis, then you may benefit from medications that are effective in increasing BMD. One popular class of drugs that decreases bone breakdown is bisphosphonates. Bisphosphonates can be prescribed as oral drugs (alendronate, ibandronate, risedronate) or as intravenous medications (pamidronate or zoledronic acid). Intravenous medications may be more effective than oral medications and are only given once every few months. Bisphosphonates are very effective but have side effects. Oral bisphosphonates are associated with stomach upset and heartburn. Intravenous bisphosphonates are associated with flu-like symptoms that improve with continued dosing. Bisphosphonates are also rarely associated with osteonecrosis of the jaw, a condition in which a section of the jawbone fails to heal, typically after a tooth is pulled. Alternatives to bisphosphonates used for osteoporosis include calcitonin, selective estrogen receptor modulators (SERMs), and parathyroid hormone or denosumab, but have not yet been widely used in MD. All of these medications have been shown to reduce the risk of fracture and have their own list of side effects.

Tayjus' Comment:

In this regard, I have followed most of the standards of care. Every day I take calcium supplements and a multivitamin that contains calcium and vitamin D. I also eat a lot of leafy greens and eat at least one serving of yogurt per day. As far as weight, I have made an effort to not be overweight and believe that I have been able to maintain a healthy weight through portion control. Finally, I have now received two doses of bisphosphonates. I have dealt with several side effects of bisphosphonates such as flu-like symptoms, but they have not been that bad.

Lilleen's Comment:

I work on bone density through aquatic therapy and PT. Now that I primarily use a scooter or wheelchair, I try to stand several times a day for as long as I can. Eating healthy and keeping my weight under control is also important.

56. How much vitamin D should I take?

Vitamin D is essential for the health of several tissues and organs in the body including bone, muscle, and the immune system. Vitamin D is required to deposit calcium into bone, and insufficient vitamin D is connected to osteoporosis.

Vitamin D is made in the skin when it is exposed to UV rays from sunlight. It is possible for some people to get enough vitamin D from the sun if they live in sunny locations. However, people who live far from the equator likely are not exposed to enough UV rays during the winter months to produce vitamin D. Sunscreen, which is important to reduce the risk of skin cancer, also, unfortunately, blocks UV rays, as does clothing. Older individuals and dark-skinned people produce less vitamin D in the skin.

Some foods such as milk and cereals are fortified with vitamin D. Fatty fish such as salmon, mackerel, and sardines contain vitamin D. Still, many people are not getting enough and are deficient, and, for them, the best option is to take supplements. Ask your physician to check your vitamin D level and suggest the correct level of supplementation, as the amount that is appropriate depends on what your current level is to start with. For people in the normal range, it may be recommended that you take as little as 400 International Units (IU) each day; or, you may need as much as 50,000 IU once a week for a few weeks if you are severely deficient. Most people do not need more than 4000 IU per day to maintain levels in the normal range. There may be side effects of taking too much vitamin D. High doses of vitamin D have been associated with high levels of calcium in the blood and some, but not all studies, suggest that high doses of vitamin D increase the risk of kidney stones. Vitamin D toxicity is extremely rare but has symptoms of nausea, vomiting, weakness, loss of appetite, and frequent urination. In general, vitamin D supplementation is very safe and is a good idea for people with MD who are at risk of low bone density.

57. I've had a fracture—now what?

Fractures can happen from a fall or from minimal trauma due to osteoporosis. They are not only painful but can be disabling. Signs that you may have had a fracture include pain, bruising, swelling, or deformity. Midline back pain may indicate a vertebral fracture.

If you suspect that you have suffered a fracture, you should head to an emergency department. You should ask the doctors there to speak with your neuromuscular team about your condition and plans for treatment. You will be seen by an orthopedic surgeon either that day or in a follow-up appointment shortly thereafter.

If you have suffered a fracture of a leg bone and you were walking prior to the fracture, the goal will be to get you up walking as soon as possible so that you do not lose this ability from immobility and muscle atrophy. For this reason, you may wish to opt for a surgical intervention, which often decreases the amount of time your broken leg must be immobilized. Weight-bearing casts are another possibility, depending on the fracture and your amount of residual strength. If your leg is casted, then it is important that the cast includes a straight knee and neutral ankle to reduce the risk of contracture formation. Vertebral fractures do not typically have surgical or casting solutions.

If you have suffered a vertebral fracture or long bone fracture from minimal trauma, then you may benefit from intravenous bisphosphonates. This class of drugs has been shown to improve the vertical height of collapsed vertebrae, reduce the pain associated with fracture, and reduce future fracture risk. An endocrinologist would prescribe this drug.

Fat embolism syndrome (see Question 41) is a rare medical emergency that occurs when a bone is fractured (usually a long bone). Fat from the bone marrow makes its way into the bloodstream where it can occlude blood vessels such as in the lung and brain leading to shortness of breath and confusion. Suspected fat embolism syndrome requires immediate intervention.

A fracture is a stressful event. If you are taking high doses of corticosteroids for MD and have adrenal insufficiency, you will need to take a stress dose of your prescribed steroids for about 24 hours after the fracture. If you require surgery for the fracture, please inform the anesthesiologist of the concern of adrenal insufficiency, as this also requires additional steroid administration to safely maintain your blood pressure through the surgery and recovery process.

It is important to continue what activity you can after a fracture. This may take the form of continued physical therapy with some limitations due to the fracture, stretching of the unaffected limbs, or simple range-of-motion exercises. You will need physical therapy to help regain function after your fracture has healed.

Tayjus' Comment:

As far as fractures go, I have fractured my distal tibia, my shoulder, and several vertebrae. When I broke my tibia, I did not need surgery to treat it. I was still walking at the time, so it was a big change to not be able to walk, and the concern was would I be able to get back to weight bearing and walking. I fortunately did not need to be casted. I was given a healing boot to wear, but the standard black boot issued was too heavy. We were able to get a fitted healing boot from my orthotist and this worked much better. I also had additional PT and aqua therapy. After all of this, I was able to return to weight bearing and walking, albeit I could now only walk short distances. At that point, I decided to start using a wheelchair, but I would walk a little to use the bathroom or transfer into chair or bed. When I broke my shoulder, I did not require a cast but started using a sling. That was able to heal normally. Finally, for the vertebral fractures, I started taking vitamin D and calcium, and eventually, bisphosphonates.

Vicky's Comment:

It's hard to imagine how compromised the bones of our boys are, due to prolonged use of steroids and the weakened muscles. Our son had multiple fractures in a period of 9 months and most of them were from minimum movements like transferring and being in a car on a bumpy road. Careful handling and movement are imperative to avoid any chance of injury or fracture.

PART NINE

Mental Health

What should I do if I'm depressed or anxious?

What is the purpose of a neuropsychological evaluation?

Are there support groups?

More . . .

58. What should I do if I'm depressed or anxious?

Living with MD is stressful and can lead to depression and anxiety. Symptoms of depression include prolonged sadness or unexplained tearfulness, loss of interest in regular activities, difficulty sleeping, loss of appetite, fatigue, feelings of worthlessness, and social withdrawal. Anxiety can manifest as excessive worrying, feeling agitated, restlessness, fatigue, difficulty concentrating, irritability, and difficulty sleeping. You may have some but not all of these symptoms and still be suffering from depression or anxiety.

It is important that you tell your healthcare professional about your symptoms. Your doctor may refer you to a licensed mental health therapist. A therapist may be a social worker, psychologist, or psychiatrist. It is important that you feel comfortable with your therapist, and it can take one or more tries to find the right person for you.

Cognitive behavioral therapy (CBT)

A therapy method aimed to challenge and change distorted thoughts and unhelpful behaviors.

Acceptance commitment therapy (ACT)

A therapy method based on accepting reality and opening up to unpleasant feelings.

There are many goals for mental health therapy that can contribute to treating depression and anxiety. This includes exploring self-esteem in relation to medical diagnosis, increasing social engagement and decreasing isolation, building healthy relationships, working toward a place of acceptance regarding having a chronic medical diagnosis, focusing on values and goals and how to reach them, managing behaviors by handling ongoing stress, frustration, and anger and teaching coping and relaxation techniques.

A couple of therapy methods have proven helpful for depression and anxiety: **cognitive behavioral therapy (CBT)** and **acceptance commitment therapy (ACT)**. CBT aims to challenge and change distorted thoughts and unhelpful behaviors. With the help of a therapist, individuals will identify harmful thoughts, assess whether they are accurate depictions of reality, and, if they are not, employ strategies to challenge and overcome them. Conversely, in ACT, the individual does not work to challenge or stop unwanted thoughts but rather to open up to unpleasant feelings, learn not to overreact to them, and learn not to avoid situations where they are invoked. A key component of ACT is values clarification, in which the therapist and individual work to increase awareness of any values that may have a bearing on lifestyle decisions and actions. Both CBT and ACT are appropriate for children and adults.

Sometimes, talk therapy is not enough to alleviate depression and anxiety. Your doctor may prescribe one or more medications to help with your symptoms. Medications for depression include selective serotonin reuptake inhibitors (SSRIs), serotonin and norepinephrine reuptake inhibitors (SNRIs), tricyclic antidepressants (TCAs) and drugs with unique mechanisms such as bupropion and trazadone. Medications for anxiety include SSRIs, TCAs, benzodiazepines, and drugs with unique mechanisms such as buspirone. If one class of medication is not helpful to you, then another class may be. Although these medications all have their own side effects, they can be very effective at relieving symptoms and restoring quality of life.

Tayjus' Comment:

I have at times found myself very frustrated with the limitations created by DMD, especially when it came to accessibility. I never really felt this until college, when I began to feel that I had limitations that prevented me from doing all the same things as my peers. While I was aware that a lot was possible with planning, I sometimes found myself only thinking of my limitations. Often issues with having to depend on personal care attendants made me frustrated, as well as knowing that this was always a piece I had to deal with. The other main source of unhappiness was inaccessibility preventing me from socializing. While I am living independently with the help of personal care attendants and am employed, I do find myself limited socially. I feel isolated sometimes, and sometimes find myself frustrated when I look at peers.

Colin's Comment:

Ever since I was first diagnosed with MD when I was 26, I have struggled with some symptoms of depression, which were even apparent to those around me. For many years after I was diagnosed, I was in denial and desperately trying to act as if there was nothing wrong with me. Depression and fear can either motivate you or immobilize you. In my case it was the latter. I would spend days alone in my apartment eating junk food, watching movies, and not doing too much else. My sleeping patterns became so erratic that my days and nights were turned around and I often would stay up all night and sleep all day. This made any kind of social interaction impossible. This went on for a while, until, after several years, I processed the stages of grief until I reached acceptance. I took responsibility for my life and my actions and tried to adopt healthy lifestyle habits and ways to avoid heading down the rabbit hole again. Through personal growth and acceptance, my life has improved, and although I still struggle, depression and fear aren't controlling my life.

59. What is the purpose of a neuropsychological evaluation?

A neuropsychological evaluation should be performed when there are concerns about cognitive delays, difficulties with emotional or behavioral regulation, or concerns about social skills. Neuropsychological evaluations are given by specially trained clinical psychologists. The evaluation characterizes the cognitive, emotional, social, and academic skills of the individual and develops a plan to address these areas of functioning.

The neuropsychological evaluation takes several hours in which the individual is taken through a sequence of tests. The time the evaluation takes is dependent on the ease of the test taker and his or her degree of cooperation. Preparation is not needed nor helpful.

Neuropsychological evaluations assist in determining baseline function, assist in diagnosis of relevant disorders (such as attention deficit disorder, autism, or learning disability), describe skill patterns that impact on school or work functioning, assist in educational planning, and monitor change in functioning.

If you or your child has a MD with a risk of associated cognitive or behavioral symptoms (such as DMD or congenital DM1), the neuropsychological exam may be a very helpful tool close to diagnosis or before beginning school. Follow-up evaluations every few years can be used to monitor progress and make changes to the educational plan. Your neurologist can make an initial assessment and refer you to a neuropsychologist.

Vicky's Comment:

We had a neuropsych exam very early on, and it helped in determining any cognitive delays, but it also helped in identifying social patterns and ways in which he communicated.

In our case, our son's cognitive ability was above normal, which actually disguised a lot of the social challenges he had. This was a much bigger issue than we anticipated and has contributed to his social/emotional health through much of middle school and now high school.

60. Are there support groups?

A support group is a group of people with common experiences or concerns who provide each other with encouragement, comfort, and advice. This can be peer led or facilitated by a social worker or another professional. Support groups provide peer-to-peer support and an avenue to build connections with people who may have similar life experiences. Support groups foster relationships, connectivity, emotional support, new ideas, and problem solving.

There are support groups for MD in general and for specific subtypes of MD. Some groups are for those personally affected by MD and some are for caregivers or parents of those with MD. Some of the larger MD clinics organize support groups for their patients. Check with your neuromuscular doctor to see if there is one at your clinic.

When you first join a support group, you may be reluctant to open up about your personal situation. It is okay to begin by just listening. Hopefully with time, you will feel comfortable sharing your own experiences and getting feedback from the group. Try a support group for a few sessions to see if the group resonates with you. If not, there are so many groups, you can try another group or different format.

Here are a few of the many groups welcoming members.

FSHD Society:
The FSHD Society has local chapters and holds events including support group meetings for those with FSHD and their family members.
https://www.fshdsociety.org/connect/support-groups/

Parent Project Muscular Dystrophy:
PPMD has Connect Groups which include family mentoring, outreach and fundraising for those families with DMD or BMD. They also offer social opportunities for parents and families.
https://www.parentprojectmd.org/get-involved /connect/find-a-local-connect-group/

Muscular Dystrophy Association:
Local offices of the MDA frequently arrange support groups for those who are registered with the MDA.
https://www.mda.org/services

Myotonic:
The Myotonic sponsors support groups across the county for those with DM as well as an online support community: The Myotonic Caregivers Support Group.
https://www.myotonic.org/find-support

Online support groups:
Through Facebook, a number of online peer support groups have been established. Many of these are "closed" Facebook groups to protect privacy. Individuals must "request to join."
Some examples of Facebook forums include
"Parent Project Muscular Dystrophy Facebook Page"
"Living with Limb-Girdle Muscular Dystrophy"
"Teens with Muscular Dystrophy"

"Women living with MD"
"Guys MD"
"Spouses Fighting Against MD"
"Cure CMD"
"Duchenne and Becker teen and adult community powered by the PAC"
There are also Facebook groups for those living in various countries and in a variety of languages.

Tayjus' Comment:

I have found support groups to be very helpful! For Duchenne, I have always found a strong community in Parent Project Muscular Dystrophy and often automatically form friendships with others with DMD around my age. We can usually relate so well without a need to explain anything. Facebook made it possible to always reach out to these friends and keep up with one another's lives. Finally, through Facebook I am part of DMD groups focused on going to college and being independent, which have been so helpful to meet people like me and discuss questions with other independent adults with DMD who are now managing their own care. I am also part of a broader MD Facebook, which is also helpful to bounce off so many different questions that no one else could totally understand.

Lilleen's Comment:

Support groups can be rewarding and educational. They can also be overwhelming, depending on where you are in accepting your diagnosis. I remember going to my first one, and leaving very overwhelmed. It was months before I returned to my next one. Each time I went back, it became easier and easier. I realized I could learn from others about what I was going through that they had already dealt with.

Remember each person is on his or her own journey and just because one person finds a support group helpful, the next person may not. There are also Facebook groups, which are great for those who may or may not be able to personally attend meetings. These groups are great for meeting people or seeking advice from people who are experiencing similar challenges. However, my one recommendation is to remember these sites may not have oversight and the information may or not be correct. This is particularly true when it comes to some scientific information or medical advice. Remember to always confirm medical advice with your own medical team.

61. What is executive dysfunction?

Executive functions are cognitive abilities that concern two main areas: (1) goal-oriented skills such as planning, organization, time management, taking initiative and getting started on things, short term and working memory (keeping important information in mind while doing tasks) and (2) self-regulatory skills such as self monitoring (evaluation how you are doing in a situation and the impact you are having on others), cognitive flexibility (being able to adjust/adapt your thinking in response to changes in circumstances or unexpected events), and self-inhibition (being able to stop and think before you say or do something and controlling your emotional reactions). Executive dysfunction or executive function disorder describes the many symptoms that can occur when these functions are disabled. Examples of executive dysfunction in everyday life include persistent difficulty getting homework turned in on time, remembering to take all your books and homework home, keeping your office or

Executive functions

Cognitive abilities that involve planning and organization as well as self-regulatory skills and self-inhibition.

bedroom organized, and following complex or detailed instructions. Weaknesses in executive function can cause problems getting things done in an efficient manner. They can also affect relationships, with patterns of being argumentative and losing your temper. Executive dysfunction can affect both children and adults. It is associated with a wide range of disorders and brain injuries and is described in many with DM and DMD.

A clinical neuropsychologist can diagnose executive dysfunction through a battery of standardized tests. Testing can differentiate between normal developmental challenges, mental health issues, and executive dysfunction. The neuropsychologist may make recommendations to the school if the individual is a child or to the workplace if the individual is an adult. Success in school and at work can be severely impaired in the setting of executive dysfunction.

Some strategies to coping with executive dysfunction include using calendars, diaries, or electronic devices to plan your day. Make schedules and look at them several times a day. When planning your day or an activity, divide the activity into manageable parts that can be accomplished and checked off. For example, if you have a paper due in school by the end of the week, plan what sections you will write each day and stick to your schedule. Prepare a weekly routine for tasks such as shopping, washing, exercise, etc. Knowing that, for example, on Tuesdays you are scheduled to go to the gym, makes it more likely that you will stick to this plan. Use external motivation such as being accountable to others at work, school, and home to reinforce accomplishing goals.

There are no specific medications for executive dysfunction. Many individuals, however, have found benefit from dopamine agonists (e.g., stimulants) and less commonly, antagonists (e.g., neuroleptics). Stimulants work quickly, and you will be able to see improvements rapidly if the medication is working for you. There are some downsides to stimulants, including the fact that you have to let them wear off at the end of the day in order to go to sleep, they are appetite suppressants and can lead to weight loss, and they can make people irritable. If irritability is a side effect, you can usually find a different stimulant that doesn't cause this.

Colin's Comment:

When I was first diagnosed with MD, I had no idea that the disease could affect cognitive processes. Of course, once I found out about executive dysfunction, some of the problems I've had in the past, especially with school, made more sense. I had lots of problems in both high school and college (which coincided with the onset of MD) with turning in homework and assignments on time, concentrating on work rather than leisure activities, and even showing up for classes. Although issues with executive function explains the cause of these difficulties, it doesn't make the emotional effects of them any easier to handle. I suffered lack of self-esteem for years. I thought that there was something wrong with me, that I was defective. To make things even worse, I had no energy or motivation to do anything. I use a stimulant now called modafinil. It has been very helpful to make me more alert, motivated, and able to stay on task. I think that the benefits of stimulants outweigh the risks, which can be mitigated as long as you are careful. Knowing the causes, effects, and strategies to combat executive dysfunction, I have been better able to cope with it. It remains a daily challenge.

62. What is obsessive–compulsive disorder?

Obsessive–compulsive disorder

A mental health disorder that involves unwanted intrusive thoughts, images, or urges that frequently cause anxiety coupled with a repetitive behavior designed to reduce psychological distress or discomfort.

Obsessive–compulsive disorder (OCD) is a mental health disorder that can affect both children and adults. An obsession refers to unwanted intrusive thoughts, images, or urges that frequently cause anxiety. A compulsion is a repetitive behavior designed to reduce psychological distress or discomfort. These behaviors are used to mitigate obsessive thoughts. OCD is defined as a disorder because it interferes with quality of life. The incidence of OCD is higher in DMD than the general population.

Common initial symptoms include difficulty with changes in routine, repetitive behaviors, and organizational compulsions. Other common symptoms of OCD include germ phobia and contamination fears. Many children with OCD require a very specific bedtime routine. An example is a boy who has a 1- to 2-hour bedtime routine in which he needs to lie in a specific way in bed, his clothing needs to be adjusted in a certain way, and doors and windows need to be checked multiple times. If these things are not done, he has significant anxiety and distress. Once they are done, the feeling of discomfort goes away temporarily, but the need for compulsive behaviors is reinforced. Many children with DMD don't have full-fledged OCD, but they are in more of a gray area: their compulsions are not exactly the same every time (as is true for OCD) but can shift from day to day and can result in the child being very particular about things.

OCD can be disabling. It is frequently associated with anxiety, depression, and ADHD. Luckily, there are effective treatments for OCD. Cognitive behavioral therapy (see Question 58) has been used successfully in many individuals. Exposure and response prevention, a technique where the individual is gradually introduced to the threat and then taught to avoid the compulsion is another approach. Finally, medications such as SSRIs can be helpful. A combination of therapy and medication may work best.

63. Would a service animal be helpful?

A service animal can be of great assistance to an individual with MD and can facilitate independence. As defined by the Americans with Disabilities Act (ADA), a **service animal** is a dog that has been individually trained to do work or perform tasks for an individual with a disability. The task(s) performed by the dog must be directly related to the person's disability.

> **Service animal**
> As defined by the Americans with Disabilities Act, a dog trained to perform specific functions or behaviors that aid an individual with disabilities.

There are many types of service dogs individually trained for specific disabilities. These include, for example, Seizure Response Dogs, Visual Assistance Dogs, and Hearing Dogs. Of particular relevance to those with MD are Brace/Mobility Support Dogs and Wheelchair Assistance Dogs.

A Brace/Mobility Support Dog provides bracing or counterbalancing to an individual who has balance issues due to a disability. The service dog frequently wears a harness which the individual can hold onto when walking or when trying to get up. Brace/Mobility Support Dogs can perform other tasks such as retrieving objects, opening and closing doors, and turning on and off light switches. They are trained to alert others in an emergency, such as a fall.

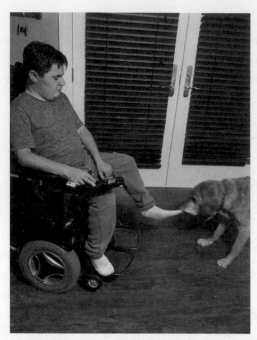

Figure 10 A service dog assists an individual with DMD by removing his sock.

Wheelchair Assistance Dogs (**Figure 10**) are trained to perform tasks for those using a wheelchair. Wheelchair Assistance Dogs are trained to adjust an individual's posture by helping to return a slumped individual back to an upright posture, place an arm back on an armrest that has fallen, or raise or lower adjustable footrests. They can help with transfers on and off the wheelchair. Wheelchair Assistance Dogs can also perform other tasks such as retrieving objects, opening and closing doors, and turning on and off light switches. Similar to Brace/Mobility Support Dogs, they are trained to alert others in case of an emergency.

Several foundations train and provide service dogs for those with disabilities. Many of these do so free of charge. It is also possible for you to train a dog yourself. However, the training is extensive and frequently lasts a couple years. After this professional training, the dog and individual with disability are brought together and the individual learns to manage the service dog's behavior, to direct the dog to respond to commands it has learned, and to assume responsibility for maintaining the health and well-being of the dog.

The ADA mandates that service animals are allowed in all public places including schools, workplace, restaurants, theaters, etc., with a few exceptions, including houses of worship and airplanes. You cannot be asked to show a certificate for your service animal or to describe your disability. You can be asked (1) is the dog a service animal required because of a disability? and (2) what work or task has the dog been trained to perform? To learn more about your rights and responsibilities as they pertain to a service animal, see https://www.ada.gov/regs2010/service_animal_qa.html.

Service dogs can perform a multitude of tasks enhancing independence and safety. They are also an emotional support. Bred specifically to be calm and relaxed, they can decrease anxiety and stress. Service dogs are an additional responsibility but can greatly enhance quality of life.

Vicky's Comment:

We got our service dog when our son was 8 years old. Looking back, this may have been a few years too early to actually assist with physical tasks, but she definitely provided friendship and companionship, which to this day has provided intrinsic value beyond words. Having a service dog is, in my opinion, one of the greatest gifts you can give a child with MD. In addition to the obvious physical benefits of picking things up, opening and closing doors, and switching lights on and off, this companion offers the kind of loyal friendship you only realize exists after you've experienced it. There is a pretty intense screening process for a service dog, but it is well worth the time and effort.

PART TEN

Pain and Fatigue

How can I treat my pain?

What can I do about fatigue?

What is palliative care?

More . . .

64. How can I treat my pain?

A large proportion of individuals with MD suffer from pain. There are multiple different types and causes of pain, but it is common for individuals with MD to experience musculoskeletal pain. The causes are not entirely clear but most likely are the result of the imbalance of musculature and the strain that is put on some muscles to compensate for other, weaker muscles. Pain reduces one's ability to engage in normal activities, leads to social isolation, and overall decreases quality of life.

You should discuss any sources of pain with your healthcare providers at every visit. Your physicians will want to make sure that you don't have a concomitant injury or ailment resulting in pain (such as back pain that is the result of a vertebral fracture). They will want to make sure that any equipment you use fits well and that your bed is supportive. They may prescribe physical therapy for gentle strengthening exercises, range-of-motion exercises, and evaluation of seating and posture.

If your pain is localized to only a discreet area, you may benefit from a lidocaine patch. An adhesive patch with local anesthesia is applied to the skin overlying the painful region. Up to three patches can be used at one time. Lidocaine patches are helpful for mild, defined areas of pain.

For more widespread or moderate to severe pain, there are several different classes of oral medications to consider. Your primary care physician, neurologist, or a pain specialist can prescribe these. One of the most effective classes of medications for musculoskeletal pain in MD is nonsteroidal anti-inflammatory medications (NSAIDs). Prescription doses of over-the-counter NSAIDs (e.g., ibuprofen) or prescription NSAIDs may be necessary to adequately treat pain. NSAIDs should be used cautiously in those who are also taking corticosteroids and carry risks of gastritis, gastric ulcer, and bleeding.

Antidepressants are another class of drugs that are helpful for musculoskeletal pain. SSRIs, specifically duloxetine, and less commonly tricyclic antidepressants are frequently effective. Other medications include gabapentin, carbamazepine, and mexiletine. Each of these medications has its own side effects and risks, which your doctor should explain to you.

Opioids are very effective analgesics. Opioids are frequently one of the last medications to be tried for MD. This is because individuals with MD frequently suffer from chronic pain, and chronic treatment with opioids brings the risk of dependency and abuse. Other risks of using opioids in MD include respiratory depression and severe constipation. However, if other attempts at pain management are unsuccessful, opioids can be considered with close monitoring.

There are also alternatives to medications that bring relief to some with MD. These include physical therapy with stretching, massage therapy, acupuncture, and transcutaneous electrical nerve stimulation (TENS). TENS uses small electrical impulses delivered through your skin, which causes your body to release natural pain killers called endorphins. TENS cannot be used in individuals with pacemakers or defibrillators. While some individuals prefer these alternatives to taking medications, others use them in conjunction with medications for greater benefit or to reduce the overall dose of medication required to treat pain.

It is important that you communicate clearly with your doctor about any pain that you are having and whether the treatments that you are prescribed are helpful. It may be necessary for you to try one, two, or more different medications or combinations before you find relief. However, with good communication and some effort, you and your doctor should be able to arrive at a solution to adequately treat your pain.

Tayjus' Comment:

Over the years, I have had various kinds of pain, and fortunately I have not had too many issues with pain recently. When I transitioned into using a wheelchair full time, I did find myself in a lot of hip pain, and it was quite challenging. I tried heating pads but they never really helped. When I started college, I had a lot of hip pain for around 3 months. It turned out that using a shower bench rather than a shower chair was causing this pain. After that I finally got a fitted specialized shower chair, and this made the difference. In some cases, the pain was due to underlying issues with bone density, which resulted in some compression fractures. I have also found PT and keeping flexible to be the key to prevent any sudden pain.

Lilleen's Comment:

How I treated my pain over the years has depended on whether it's muscular or not. I have both muscular and joint pain (hips, elbows, hands). Before transitioning to a scooter/ wheelchair full time, I had more muscular pain. That pain was caused from overexerting muscles from walking or standing for long periods of time. Now my pain is primarily joint pain in my hips. I usually take naproxen for the pain when I feel the need. However, in the past I have also received steroid injections in my hip. Although this treatment is very intrusive, it can help eliminate the pain for weeks if not months. For muscular pain, I treat it several ways: massages, TENS device, essential oils, heating pad. What has helped the most is doing PT and aquatic therapy.

65. What can I do about fatigue?

Fatigue is a major symptom for most MDs. It can lead to withdrawal from activities, detracting from work and home life. It can be disabling.

You should discuss your fatigue with your neuromuscular physician or primary care provider. He or she should check for other medical causes of fatigue such as anemia or hypothyroidism. These conditions can be treated. Your neuromuscular physician will want to ask you about your sleep, whether you are getting enough hours and if the quality is good. A sleep study may be prescribed to evaluate for obstructive sleep apnea (OSA) or other sleep disorder. OSA is a condition in which the individual has multiple mini-awakenings in the night due to obstruction of the air passages during sleep. These mini-awakenings keep the individual from going into the deepest restorative sleep. OSA is treatable with CPAP (see Question 37), and treatment can greatly relieve symptoms of fatigue and sleepiness. This is particularly important for those who are overweight or have DM, both of which increase the risk of OSA.

Your neuromuscular physician, primary care provider, or social worker will also want to screen you for depression. One of the main symptoms of depression is fatigue along with loss of interest in activities, difficulty sleeping, loss of appetite, and loss of libido. Depression is treatable, including mental health therapy and medications (see Question 58).

If you and your physician have addressed all other physical and mental causes of fatigue and you are still having difficulties, then there are a couple of options for treatment. The first recommendation would be to try energy conservation therapy. In this technique, you learn how to minimize muscle fatigue, joint stress, and pain. This therapy is usually conducted with a physical or occupational therapist. Some recommendations include spacing out activities throughout the day, performing the activities that take more energy during the time of day when you have more energy or are feeling your best, use of AFOs (Question 23) or assistive devices, implementation of breaks throughout the day as needed to maximize energy, and simplifying tasks to make them easier and more approachable to do. This is only a partial list of energy conservation techniques that the OT or PT can provide after discussing your activities. Many people find energy conservation therapy very useful in teaching them how to conserve their energy for those activities that are most important to them.

A second-line option for treatment is the use of a stimulant. Medications such as modafinil or dextroamphetamine are extremely effective against fatigue. They have dependency and abuse potential and should be prescribed at the lowest effective dose. They also have risks of high heart rate, mania, anorexia, headache, and irritability. It is important to take these medications early in the day so that they do not contribute to nighttime insomnia.

Fatigue is a common but treatable problem in those with MD. It is important to determine the cause of the fatigue and then treatment options can be considered.

Vicky's Comment:

For my son, fatigue has been an issue in school, particularly towards the end of the day. Though difficult to get used to at first, using the BIPAP at night really helped with sleep quality, which showed up as having more energy during the day. Having an IEP or a 504 Plan in school can also help by providing accommodations that allow kids to have support at times it is most needed.

66. Should I push through my pain and fatigue to increase strength and stamina?

My experience with those with MD is that they are strong in spirit. They minimize their disability and push themselves to achieve their goals. It is not surprising, therefore, that I am frequently asked how hard one should push oneself.

A certain amount of perseverance through discomfort is almost certainly necessary for those with MD in order to carry out the tasks of daily living. However, pushing through pain and fatigue as a way to increase strength and stamina, for example in physical therapy, should be avoided. Pain is a useful measure of the body's ability to function. Ignoring these cues can lead to excessive strain on muscle with resulting damage. Similarly, when you continue to exert yourself when greatly fatigued, you are more prone to falls and injury. Stop when you are in pain or fatigued.

Tayjus' Comment:

I do not believe one should unnecessarily push through pain and fatigue especially if there is a way of doing things better.

Living with MD means that one needs to accept when things have become harder. Sometimes it may mean starting to use a wheelchair full time. When you live with MD, you often want to push yourself to achieve your goals. This is great, but it should not be at the cost of your own health and well-being.

67. What is palliative care?

Many people are unfamiliar with what palliative care means or can offer. Palliative care is a model of care that focuses on the relief of suffering and improvement of quality of life across the spectrum of illness. It is a holistic approach, integrating emotional, psychosocial, spiritual, developmental, and existential needs of patients and families and providing relief from physical pain and symptoms. Palliative care is often and mistakenly viewed as only relevant to patients who are nearing the end-of-life. However, the goals of palliative care—to relieve suffering and improve quality of life—are appropriate for all stages of MD. Palliative care can include pain and other symptom management, case management, counseling about decision-making, attention to ethical issues, mental health care, respite care, pastoral care, advance directives planning, and other supportive services.

Some worry that to embrace palliative care is to abandon hope and disease-modifying treatments. This is not true. Palliative care can be offered in parallel—not instead of—other forms of treatment. When palliative care is reframed as support for maximizing quality of life, it provides enormous benefit. Benefits include guidance in decision making for major medical interventions (i.e., scoliosis surgery, tracheostomy); encouragement of the individual and the family to focus on quality of life issues; and assistance with care coordination and pain and symptom management. An essential element of palliative care is to anticipate stressors and plan in advance to incorporate the wishes of the individual and family as serious or life-threatening problems develop. Individuals and families who have adequately explored their preferences involving changes in function are more able to adjust to these changes.

Palliative care is often provided by a multidisciplinary team that frequently includes a specialty-trained palliative care doctor, nurse, chaplain, and social worker. As such, palliative care is not integrated in many MD clinics. It is worth asking if your clinic can make a referral to palliative care. If not, your clinic may have many features of palliative care that it can offer you with your neuromuscular doctor serving as the coordinator of care.

PART ELEVEN

Surgeries

When is scoliosis surgery recommended?

Should I get tendon releases?

Who would benefit from scapular fixation surgery?

More . . .

68. When is scoliosis surgery recommended?

Scoliosis is the lateral side-to-side curvature of the spine. It is common in some MDs, such as pediatric-onset LGMD, FSHD, and DMD. Scoliosis usually affects adolescents who are using a wheelchair full time. Long-term corticosteroid use has greatly reduced the need for scoliosis surgery.

Untreated scoliosis can become disfiguring. Scoliosis surgery can improve comfort and seating tolerance, cosmetic appearance, and may improve or stabilize respiratory function. Without scoliosis surgery, there is risk of skin breakdown and pain from the ribs rubbing against the iliac crest in the concavity of the scoliosis.

The surgery is lengthy and complex. Stainless steel or titanium rods are placed on either side of the spine and connected via wires or screws and hooks. The vertebrae in the curve are straightened and connected to each other and the rods. The vertebrae eventually fuse together.

The surgery is not without risks. Complications may include postoperative pneumonia, wound breakdown, surgical wound infection, need for blood transfusion, failure of the spine to fuse, collapsed lung, and chronic pain.

The decision when to operate is complex because all patients do not progress at the same rate. Early surgery is indicated for those who have rapid progression of their scoliosis or those whose respiratory and cardiac function is such that later surgery would put them at greater operative risk. Previous recommendations were for spinal instrumentation and fusion in those whose spinal curve was >20 degrees, were prepubertal, and were not on glucocorticoids because progression of the curve was expected. However, now many surgeons wait until the spinal curve is 40 to 50 degrees in recognition of improved perioperative management and to avoid having to make the decision too early. Determination of progression of scoliosis from serial X-rays dictates surgery. In nonambulatory teenagers with MD, a spinal X-ray should evaluate scoliosis every 6–12 months depending on rate of progression. A referral to an orthopedic surgeon should occur when the spinal curve is >20 degrees.

Following surgery, the individual with MD will be hospitalized for a few days and then most likely transferred to a rehabilitation facility for a few weeks. There he or she will work extensively with PT and OT to relearn how to do things with a straight spine. Some functions may be recovered, but some may be lost, including the hand-to-mouth function. The taller trunk may also affect reaching low.

Scoliosis surgery is a significant surgery with risks and long rehabilitation requirements. However, for those who have rapidly progressive and severe scoliosis, surgery has been shown to increase quality of life.

69. Should I get tendon releases?

Sometimes daily stretching and wearing nighttime AFOs do not do enough to keep contractures from forming. In patients with CMD, pediatric LGMD, BMD, or DMD, for example, tight Achilles tendons can present with toe walking and an inability to place the heel on the ground. This can make the work of walking harder. However, toe walking can also be a compensation for hip and quadriceps weakness. It's essential to know when it is helpful to do tendon releases (also known as heel cord tenotomy, heel cord release, or Achilles tendon releases) versus when it can actually be detrimental to function.

Tenotomy is decided on a case-by-case basis. It is important to discuss this option with an experienced orthopedic surgeon in addition to your neurologist. Tenotomy is indicated when the contractures are out of proportion to the weakness and are leading to destabilization of the gait. It is not indicated when the child has extensive weakness and is using toe walking as a compensatory mechanism.

The surgery is a small incision at each heel to cut and lengthen the tendon. Following surgery, it is important that an ambulatory child with MD begins walking immediately again. This can be done in walking casts. After casts are removed, he or she should wear nighttime AFOs and resume stretching so that contractures do not re-form.

Tenotomy is also sometimes performed on older non-ambulatory individuals. When contractures at this stage become severe, it is hard to rest the foot on the wheelchair footplates and wear shoes. Tenotomy can alleviate those problems but requires the use of AFOs to keep the contractures from re-forming. Many non-ambulatory individuals decide that they are not going to fight contractures at their ankles once they are no longer walking. This is a reasonable choice, and the decision to get tenotomy at this stage is one of individual preference.

Tenotomy

A surgical procedure to cut and lengthen the tendon to relieve tendon contracture.

Tendon releases of hamstrings and hips are generally not recommended as these contractures readily re-form without the ability to brace.

An alternative to tenotomy is serial casting. Serial casting uses a series of casts to stretch soft tissue for an extended period of time. This is done by applying a series of casts to gradually improve the child's range of motion. The number of casts depends on the degree of contracture but averages three casts worn for 1 week each. The child is able to continue to ambulate with cast boots. Similar to tenotomy, it is important to follow up serial casting with daily stretches and AFOs to prevent contractures from re-forming. Serial casting avoids potential risks of tenotomies including over lengthening, infection, scarring, and anesthesia risks.

In summary, tenotomy or serial casting are interventions to combat the development of contractures. The timing of the intervention is critical so as not to hasten functional decline. An experienced orthopedic surgeon can help you make this decision.

70. Who could benefit from scapular fixation surgery?

Scapular fixation is a surgery for those who have difficulty lifting their arms due to "winging" or protrusion of their scapula or shoulder blade from their back (see Figure 11). This is seen primarily in FSHD but can also be seen in LGMD2A (LGMDR1). In those who have preserved upper arm muscle strength (i.e., the deltoids), fixing the scapula surgically to the rib cage allows the deltoids to do their job of lifting the arm more easily. Typically, individuals can get 90 degrees or slightly

Scapular fixation

A surgery in which the scapula is surgically fixed to the rib cage allowing greater range of motion for some individuals with scapular winging.

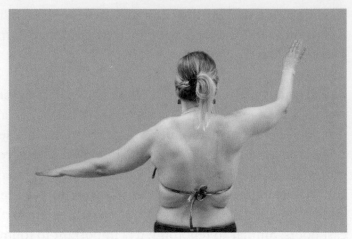

Figure 11 Individual with FSHD who has scapular winging on the left and scapular fixation on the right with improved range of motion.

greater range of motion after scapular fixation. Along with this functional improvement, individuals have reported an improvement in shoulder pain and in aesthetics after scapular fixation.

Scapular fixation is a major surgery and requires general anesthesia. An incision is made close to the border of the scapula and the scapula is fixed to the rib cage with wires. A bone graft, such as from the hip bone, is used to cement the process.

For the first six weeks after scapular fixation, the patient is asked to wear a sling and not use the arm. After that, rehabilitative physical therapy is undertaken for a period of 3 months, during which there is gradual increased activity of the shoulder. It is important to be diligent with therapy.

There are risks to scapular fixation including the risks of general anesthesia, infection, pain, bleeding, failure to heal ("nonunion"), and stiff shoulder. However, many surgeries yield a good outcome with resolved winging and improved contour and function.

Successful scapular fixations involve the right patient and the right surgeon. The right patient is one who has limited overhead arm motion due to scapular winging but has good rotator cuff muscle and deltoid strength. This can be assessed by the surgeon doing a manual compression test in which the scapula is pushed against the rib cage while the arm is being extended. The right patient also needs to be in good general health and motivated to follow postoperative rehabilitation instructions. Equally important is selection of the right surgeon. Scapular fixation surgeries are done infrequently, and it is crucial to find a surgeon who has experience doing them and has had good outcomes. Talk to your neurologist for recommendations and talk to other patients about their experience.

Lilleen's Comment:

Deciding if scapula fixation surgery is right for you is not as easy as a simple yes or no answer. You must weigh the benefits against the risks. Don't underestimate the procedure; this is a major surgery. You will need help for several days if not weeks after surgery. For me, the decision to have the surgery was totally for increased mobility and better function of my right arm. I could not lift my right arm up to brush my teeth, wash or brush my hair, or grab anything out from a cabinet. My surgeon told me I was an ideal candidate for the surgery after examining me and my muscle strength. She showed me by stabilizing my shoulder manually with her hands how I would benefit. You may want to talk with others who have had the surgery. Find out where they had their surgery and then, if possible, meet with a couple of those surgeons. Make sure you have an experienced surgeon who has done this surgery many times and has had great success. For me this surgery was life changing in a very positive way.

71. What is ptosis repair?

In some of the MDs, including DM and OPMD, a drooping of the upper eyelids, called **ptosis,** can occur. Muscles of eyelid opening and closure become weak in these diseases. Ptosis is more than a cosmetic defect, as the drooping eyelid can obscure vision in individuals with MD. When affected by MD, the levator muscle that opens the eye and lifts the upper eyelid loses some of its function, and the upper eyelid droops. If ptosis is blocking the vision, and the levator muscle still has moderate function, a surgery can be performed to tighten the levator tendon and is referred to as a levator advancement or levator resection. If the levator muscle function is poor, surgery to correct the ptosis is called a frontalis sling. In this surgery, the elevating function of the frontalis muscle, the forehead muscle that lifts the eyebrows, is used to lift the eyelids. Both procedures are typically covered by medical insurance if the vision is being compromised by the drooping eyelids. Ptosis repair surgery is different from blepharoplasty surgery, which removes excess eyelid skin. If the excess eyelid skin is not blocking the vision, a blepharoplasty is considered cosmetic and not covered by medical insurance. Blepharoplasty can be combined with a levator advancement procedure.

It is important to find an **oculoplastic surgeon** with experience in MD for these procedures. Risks of surgery include infection, dry eyes, and inability to completely close the eyes. The procedure is generally done in an

Ptosis

Drooping of the eyelid most commonly caused by weakness in the levator muscle.

Oculoplastic surgeon

A surgeon who specializes in ophthalmologic surgery to treat disorders of the eyelids and other regions around the eye.

outpatient setting with intravenous sedation and local anesthesia and can take 1 to 2 hours. Following surgery, you may have bruising and swelling for a couple of weeks. Continued weakening in a progressive MD can lead to recurrent ptosis and the need to repeat the surgery.

72. What precautions should be taken with anesthesia?

Anesthesia risks vary depending on the type of MD, condition of the individual, and type of surgery. It is critical that you inform your surgeon and anesthesiologist about your type of MD and your cardiopulmonary status. Your neuromuscular physician, cardiologist, and pulmonologist should communicate with the surgeon and anesthesiologist about your risks. You will have a preoperative evaluation in which your heart and lung function, as well as your general health, will be evaluated.

Some types of anesthesia are associated with poor outcomes in certain MDs. Volatile or inhaled anesthetic agents and one particular skeletal muscle relaxant (succinylcholine) are associated with rhabdomyolysis (massive breakdown of muscle). Rhabdomyolysis in this setting can cause kidney damage, dangerously high serum potassium, abnormal heart rhythms, and cardiac arrest. Succinylcholine is contraindicated in any patient with MD. Volatile anesthetic agents are probably safe in some MDs (e.g., DM and FSHD) but should be avoided in others (e.g., DMD and BMD). There is very little information on volatile anesthetic agents in the LGMDs, and, for this reason, they should probably be avoided. The exception to volatile anesthetic agents is nitrous oxide, which has been shown to be safe in MDs, including DMD and BMD.

Following surgery, the individual with MD will need to be monitored closely and for an extended period of time in a postanesthesia care unit. This is because individuals with MD have a higher risk of difficulty breathing including apnea (the temporary cessation of breathing) following anesthesia and are also at risk of aspiration. An individual with MD may need to be intubated longer postoperatively or they may need to be put on noninvasive ventilatory support following removal of the breathing tube. Postoperative use of sedatives and opiates should be used cautiously and under close monitoring due to risks of difficulty breathing and aspirating.

PART TWELVE

School and Muscular Dystrophy

When should I tell the school about the diagnosis?

What are IEP and 504 Plans?

Which is a better option—private or public school?

More...

73. When should I tell the school about the diagnosis?

You may be uncertain whether the school needs to know about your child's diagnosis of MD, especially if there are few or no visible signs. You may be worried that the teacher or children will treat your child differently. It may feel like an invasion of privacy to share this information. When to discuss the diagnosis with the school is a very personal decision. However, here are a few considerations.

Even if your child is not yet clearly exhibiting any signs or symptoms of MD, you may still benefit from having another set of informed eyes on your child. Your teacher may be able to alert you if your child begins having difficulty getting up from the ground, playing on the equipment at recess, following directions, or learning. If the teacher knows what to look out for in MD, then this may help you both provide a supportive environment to help your child be successful and happy at school.

When other children understand about a child's disability, they are more likely to be protective and inclusive.

As soon as you suspect or receive feedback that your child is struggling in school or that his motor function is impacting school participation or performance, you will want to disclose the diagnosis. This is necessary for your child to receive accommodations such as through an Individual Education Plan or IEP as well as a 504 Plan (see Question 74). It is also helpful for the teacher, school, and classmates to understand your child's actions and behaviors in the context of this medical condition.

Foundations such as Parent Project Muscular Dystrophy (PPMD), the Muscular Dystrophy Association

(MDA), and the FSHD Society provide excellent resources for educators about MD. These guides provide information on the manifestations of MD, common problems and solutions for students with MD, suggestions for IEP and 504 Plan accommodations, and the social and emotional needs of children with MD, among others. There are many resources to help you with this process. See Appendix B for useful websites.

The school is legally mandated to keep any medical information that you provide them confidential. However, you may want to share information about MD with your child's class. This could be done through a variety of ways: speaking to the class yourself, having your child speak to the class, showing an age-appropriate PPMD video, or having your local MDA representative visit the class. Advantages to sharing with the class is that it takes the mystery out of differences that classmates may have already been observing, allows you the opportunity to point out ways in which the child is like classmates, reduces resentment for accommodations, and encourages the classmates to act compassionately. Research shows that when other children understand about a child's disability, they are more likely to be protective and inclusive. Sharing this information with classmates can literally be the difference between a good year and a bad year at school.

Although it may not be necessary to share information at diagnosis, there are several advantages to educating the school, teacher, and class about your child's MD. Remember, though, you don't have to share *everything* about your child's or family's history.

74. What are IEP and 504 Plans?

An Individual Education Plan (IEP) and a 504 Plan are created by the school and parents to detail how a student with a disability will best learn in the least restrictive environment. The IEP is guided by the Individuals with Disabilities Education Act (IDEA), which provides special educational support to a student with a disability that negatively impacts his or her ability to learn in a regular educational environment. The 504 Plan is guided by Section 504 of the Rehabilitation Act, which specifies that no one with a disability can be excluded from participating in federally funded programs including schooling. The two plans address slightly different aspects of the educational environment for a student with a disability.

To qualify for an IEP, the student must have a disability that falls under one of the 13 categories IDEA covers and, as a result of that disability, needs additional special educational support to succeed in school (https://sites.ed.gov/idea/regs/b/a/300.8). An orthopedic impairment is one such disability that may affect the educational performance of a student with MD, allowing him or her to qualify for an IEP. A student with MD may also have a specific learning disability that requires special education and qualifies for an IEP.

To qualify for a 504 Plan, the student must have a disability that affects a major life activity, such as eating, mobility, or breathing. This disability does not have to fall under one of the 13 categories covered by IDEA, and it does not need to have an educational impact. Students who do not meet criteria for an IEP but who still require some accommodations in order to fully participate in school would be candidates for a 504 Plan. Examples would be students who require medical interventions, such as seizure medications or insulin, or assistive devices, such as wheelchairs, in order to safely function in a school environment but who otherwise have no issues learning the material being taught.

The IEP process is more involved than that of a 504 Plan. An IEP must meet strict legal requirements and be constructed by a team that includes the student's parents, at least one of the student's general education teachers, at least one of the student's special education teachers, a school psychologist or other professional who can interpret evaluation results, and a district representative with authority over special education services. An IEP is a written document that will include the child's present levels of performance, via an assessment of objective baseline metrics for each area affected by the disability; measurable goals and benchmarks via descriptions of what the student is expected to accomplish within the school year with the provision of special education services and how the education system is going to track progress toward these accomplishments; a description of special education services and related services (including the time, frequency, and types of services that will be provided); and any other accommodations needed. There are more safeguards in place for an IEP than in a 504 Plan, including the necessity to notify the parents in writing of any change to the IEP and the right to "stay put" or to continue the current services while a disagreement with an IEP is being worked out. States receive additional funding for students with IEPs. An IEP is for students ages 3–21 only.

A 504 Plan has less strict rules, and the planning process does not have to include the parents. The team generally includes parents, general and special education teachers, and the school principal or, if applicable, the school's nursing staff. Unlike an IEP, a 504 Plan does not have to be a written document. It will generally include the accommodations and services designed for the student as well as the names of the persons responsible for any services and the names of the persons who will implement the plan. States do not receive funding for 504 Plans, but federal funding can be withdrawn from schools or programs that don't meet their legal duty to serve students with disabilities. Section 504 safeguards the rights of a person with disabilities throughout his or her life span.

An IEP is a better option for a student who has a disability that negatively impacts his or her ability to receive academic instruction and who would benefit from special education. A student who receives special education services is entitled to modification of curriculum, classroom accommodations, specialized instruction, and related services such as occupational therapy, physical therapy, and speech therapy. A 504 Plan is a better option for the student who is able to function well in a regular education environment with some accommodations. Both the IEP and 504 Plan should be updated annually to make sure that the student is receiving the most effective accommodations to be successful in school.

Tayjus' Comment:

During my schooling, I was under an IEP. Though I was able to function well in a regular education environment, my parents decided that I should have an IEP to ensure that I would still be able to receive PT and OT in school. My parents and I would likely still recommend an IEP to an individual even if he or she functions in a regular education environment in order to ensure he or she can receive some of these other services.

Vicky's Comment:

Both the IEP and 504 Plan are designed to help students get the resources and appropriate supports to put them on a level playing ground with their fully abled peers. From our experience, both played important roles at different times. Our son had a 504 Plan through middle school and then switched over to an IEP in high school when his needs became greater. Both provided the necessary support he required at each stage. The IEP is definitely a more enforceable plan and allows for smaller and more detailed accommodations.

Lilleen's Comment:

Having an IEP for our son allowed him to receive several services during his school year he otherwise would not have had with a 504 Plan in our school district. These included OT, PT, and speech therapy. The IEP/504 allows a child with a disability/medical issue the same opportunities and access to learning as a child without a disability. Both types of plans allow them to remain with their peers in a regular classroom environment for learning.

75. Which is a better option—private or public school?

Whether you choose a private or public school for your child is dependent on your values and financial resources, your child's abilities, and the options in your school district. Both private and public schools are required to provide accommodations to those with disabilities, but accommodations may be more limited at a private school. Public schools are required to follow the federal education laws such as IDEA that is used to design and implement an IEP (Question 74). Private schools do not have to follow these federal laws, although depending on the degree of federal funding they receive, they may be required to comply with Section 504. Private schools receiving federal funds are obligated to comply with the least restrictive environment mandate and comparable facilities requirement, provide an equal opportunity to participate in extracurricular activities, and provide minor adjustments to accommodate students with disabilities. A service plan is developed in the private school, but it can be very different from an IEP and much more limited. The number and frequency of services that are available to your child may be greater under a public school's IEP. For example, both private and public schools may offer physical therapy, but the public school may offer it once a week while the private school offers it once per month. Special education teachers need to be state certified at public schools, while this is not a requirement at private schools. Private schools also do not have the same procedural safeguards such as the right to file for due process or mediation.

Private schools generally have smaller class sizes and a higher teacher-to-student ratio. This can be helpful for any child, but particularly one with ADHD who needs redirection. Private schools may be more flexible and amenable to requests made by parents, although this is very school dependent.

Of course, public schooling is free, and private education can be quite expensive. In some circumstances, a public school district may be required to pay for private school placement. When students with learning disabilities cannot be adequately accommodated in a public school program and the child's IEP team agrees upon a private school placement, the district is responsible for paying for private schooling.

Visit the schools in your area and talk to the administrators about accommodations that they may have made for other children or what they anticipate they will make for your child. Talk to other parents whose children have attended these schools. Factor in location: Long drives or bus rides can be exhausting for a child with MD, and it is important to have friends in the area for easy playdates.

Remember to reevaluate your options every few years. What is the best fit for an elementary school child may not be the same as for a high schooler, as abilities, needs, and preferences may change.

Tayjus' Comment:

I personally believe public school is a better option, at least if you have access to a decent public school. I went through the public school system and was able to receive PT twice a week, OT once a week, and I was provided with an aide. My parents had briefly considered private school, but concluded that public school would make more sense as public schools must follow the federal education laws completely. I was fortunate in that my public school was very supportive all along and provided me with all the accommodations I needed while in school.

Vicky's Comment:

My son was diagnosed while we were international expats, and he was attending a private school overseas. Evaluations and accommodations were much harder to conduct and implement. When we moved back to the United States and discovered the legal responsibilities of public schools for kids with disabilities, it was an easy decision for us to transition to a public school. Going from a 504 Plan in second grade to now having an IEP in high school, we have been very happy with the supports in place to help my son reach his potential in school.

Colin's Comment:

Although I wasn't diagnosed with MD until I was 26, it is very possible that the struggles I had in school were due to MD. I attended both public and private schools. My three years at a small, private elementary school were really the only time in my education that I actually enjoyed. In public school in the seventh grade, things started to change. I wasn't struggling academically at first, but socially I had lots of problems. Transferring from a small, private school with an atmosphere of respect and compromise to a much larger public school was an unpleasant experience. I begged my parents to send me to a private boarding school. Some of my problems followed me, but I did better socially. One of the advantages of attending a new school was that no one knew me, so I could be whoever I wanted. I have experienced problems in both public and private schools; however, I found private school superior to public school both academically and socially.

76. What is a paraprofessional?

A paraprofessional, or paraeducator, is part of the educational team as an assistant to a teacher. The U.S. Department of Education states that the paraprofessional must have a high school diploma or equivalent and have completed two years of college study or obtained an associate's degree. They must pass an assessment demonstrating knowledge of and the ability to assist in the instruction of reading, writing, and math. Individual states or school districts may require additional certification.

Paraprofessionals may be assigned to work with a student one-on-one, in a small group, or with the entire classroom under the direction of the teacher. They may not provide instruction except under the direct supervision of the teacher. Paraprofessionals may be assigned to a student with behavioral challenges, rewarding them for good behavior and redirecting disruptive behavior. Paraprofessionals can be helpful for children with ADHD or executive dysfunction, helping them focus and stay on task. They may also be assigned to students who have physical challenges, helping with feeding, transporting, or using the bathroom.

A paraprofessional differs from an aide in that an aide does not need to have the same credentials and may only have a high school diploma and no certification. An aide may be sufficient for the needs of a child who has only physical challenges. However, a paraprofessional should be sought for behavioral or educational assistance.

A paraprofessional is assigned to work with a child as determined by his IEP or 504 Plan. The assignment is based on the student's educational need. Need is determined by evaluation of the child (either through the school or private evaluation) and through classroom observations. If you feel that your child would benefit from a one-on-one paraprofessional, think about what skills deficits and behaviors would benefit from a one-on-one and make sure they are clearly identified in the evaluation. The responsibilities and tasks of the paraprofessional need to be clearly defined in the IEP or 504 Plan.

A paraprofessional can have a profoundly positive impact on your child's school experience with improved behavior, learning, and/or assistance with ADLs. However, there are some potential risks to having a paraprofessional assigned to your child. The teacher may take less ownership of the student working with a paraprofessional. The quality of peer interactions can be diminished with an adult ever present. Finally, the use of a paraprofessional may impact the student's ability to become an independent learner. The judicious use of a paraprofessional only for times and services that are needed is critical to support the student and encourage independence.

77. What are reasonable accommodations that a school should make?

Schools are required to make reasonable accommodations according to a child's disability unless such changes would fundamentally alter the nature of the school's purpose. The accommodations that a school makes for a child with MD should ensure that he or she is safe and has the greatest opportunity to succeed in the classroom.

However, what is a reasonable accommodation is not defined by IDEA or Section 504. The accommodations that your child needs will be specific to his or her level of physical and cognitive functioning. It is therefore important to review and update the IEP/504 Plan yearly. Below are some accommodations frequently found in IEP/504 Plans for children with MD.

- Accessibility
  - Wheelchair-accessible bus
  - Curb-to-curb transportation
  - Use of ramp and elevator
  - Extra time to travel between classes
  - Buddy or aide to carry/get out books and supplies
- Assistive technology
  - Assistive technology evaluation
  - Tablet or computer
  - Recording device
  - Voice recognition software
- Classroom modifications
  - Use of a chair rather than sitting on floor
  - Supportive seating with arms to support upright posture
  - Larger desk to accommodate wheelchair or supportive chair
  - Seat at front of class
- Exam and assignment modifications
  - Extra time for exams
  - Oral exams/reports in place of written exams/reports
  - Extra time for assignments

- Condensed assignments with less writing
- Longer or more complex assignments broken into smaller segments
- Frequent breaks to conserve energy
- Extra set of books (one for home, one for school)
- Physical education and recess
  - Adaptive PE
  - Use of an indoor room to play board games during recess
- Services
  - Aide or nurse to assist with toileting
  - Physical therapy
  - Occupational therapy
  - Speech therapy
  - Paraprofessional
  - Special education

Tayjus' Comment:

School districts are legally required to make accommodations according to the child's disability, and ideally, they will do so without a fight. The school district in my town was one of the best when it came to accommodations and other towns were known to send their students to my school district. Personally, I received PT, OT, and an aide my entire time in school. In elementary school, the school even paid for a specialized supportive chair. Some of the other services I made use of were a wheelchair-accessible bus, as well as extra time. It all depends on the student, of course, but hopefully the school district will ensure that the student receives all the accommodations that he or she needs and that the school is required to provide.

Vicky's Comment:

The most beneficial accommodation for my son was extra time between classes. In middle and high school, he was allowed to leave 3 minutes earlier than the rest of the students to allow him enough time to get to his next class on time. This was very helpful also because it allowed him to move swiftly and safely through the halls without the mass rush of students that shuffled through the hallways once the dismissal bell rang. My son was also provided with a full-time paraprofessional to help with toileting, organizing books and papers, and general tasks that he could not do on his own. Other helpful accommodations included an accessible bus for school outings, a scribe, shortened homework assignments, and assistive technology like a ChromeBook laptop and voice-to-text software.

Lilleen's Comment:

As a parent, you are your child's biggest advocate. As your child gets older, it's best to encourage self advocacy. This will help as they enter into college where there is no IEP or 504 plan. However, in college the students can request accommodations through the school's disabilities office. Accommodations for our son changed throughout his 13 years of schooling. In elementary his IEP primarily focused on services like PT, OT, speech therapy, and classroom modifications. In middle school and high school, his IEP included more assistive technology, like using an iPad or laptop, extra set of books at home, copies of teacher's notes if needed for study, extra time for testing, and extended time for homework and assignments. In college, it was extended time for testing, and no penalty for a missed class.

78. What help is there for reading and writing?

Early detection and intervention for reading and/or writing difficulties are important. Difficulties in these areas are often identified and addressed through the student's school program and implementation of special services. For some individuals with MD, problems with writing speed and efficiency can begin to occur at a later age as a result of upper extremity weakness, fatigue, and impaired range of motion.

Below is a list of several supports that can assist in addressing specific identified problems in reading and/or writing. However, use of any supports should be based on your individual needs.

Reading supports may include:

- Use of text-to-speech software to see text and hear it read aloud at the same time.
- Access to PDF annotation software with text-to-speech feature
- Access to graphic organizers to take notes during reading assignments. (Consider need for instructional support when initiating implementation of this strategy.)
- Instructional support with respect to highlighting/ underlining, adding comments, and/or use of software to take notes during reading assignments
- Adjust settings within word-processing devices such as font, font size, icon size, spacing, and/or contrast
- Use of "speak selection" function on smartphone to listen to text messages and quickly read short written material

- Use of audiobook subscription service to promote access to literature at grade level in audiobook format
- Support of an oral reader to assist individual with completion of assignments in reasonable time period
- Reduce amount of visual clutter when presented with reading assignments. Consider use of line-by-line visual supports.

Writing supports may include:

Supports related to fine motor or upper extremity weakness:

- Access to handwriting tools to support physical activity (i.e., proper seating and positioning, lightweight pencil grips, proper upper extremity support)
- Adjust amount of work and/or time frame to complete assignments secondary to fatigue
- Modify/provide alternatives to writing assignments such as fill-in-the-blank statements, multiple-choice questions, or true/false format
- Offer alternatives to in-class essay assignments/tests such as giving an oral presentation or completing a take-home assignment
- Use of a scribe as needed
- Use of speech-recognition built into tablet/phone device keyboard to dictate notes, reminders, and text messages
- Allow lectures to be recorded or provide copy of outline/notes
- Implement consistent use of computer, laptop, or tablet for written assignments

- Use of word prediction software to increase the speed of typing and reduce fatigue by decreasing the number of keystrokes needed
- Use of a smaller keyboard or laptop when muscle weakness and/or limited active range of motion is present
- Alternative computer keyboard methods in the setting of progressive muscle weakness, including:
  - On-screen keyboard via mouse or alternative mouse control (including head pointing or eye gaze)
  - Use of speech-to-text software

Supports related to writing literacy and content:

- Use of electronic graphic organizers to conduct pre-writing planning
- Access to spell-check and grammar-check supports
- Access to language/grammar support software to promote language expansion
- Use of text-to-speech supports to promote awareness and independence when editing and/or provide real-time feedback while words are typed
- Access to dictionary and/or thesaurus to support understanding of words and increased vocabulary use
- Provide strategies that will support difficulties with word retrieval, including:
  - Multiple-choice or true/false question formats
  - Access to word bank
  - Assignment-specific vocabulary list

Technology is constantly changing, and available computer/software supports for more complex reading and writing difficulties continues to advance. To foster success in reading and writing, early identification of needed interventions or alternative writing access methods are important. Assistance can be sought through a student's school or therapy program. The purchase of alternative computer access equipment is not covered by insurance. Testing the equipment before purchase is beneficial and can often be done through the student's school assistive technology team or a hospital-based assistive technology program.

Vicky's Comment:

My son was always a bright and enthusiastic learner. However, we did start to notice some lag in his desire and ability to read independently. By the time he was in fourth grade, the school and I realized that he needed support due to the fact that his upper body was weakening and the simple act of holding a book had become challenging. The school was on it and extremely supportive in offering support, by way of voice-to-text writing apps, audio books, and other technology devices to keep his interest in reading alive.

79. What are treatment options for attention deficit hyperactivity disorder?

Attention deficit hyperactivity disorder (ADHD) is the most common neurobehavioral disorder of childhood and is more common in some MDs, such as DMD, BMD, and DM1, than in the general population. ADHD is marked by persistent inattention or hyperactivity/impulsivity that interferes with function. Inattention can manifest, for example, by trouble holding attention on tasks or at play, frequently losing things, or reluctance to perform tasks that required sustained mental effort over long periods of time. Children with ADHD may pay good attention to things that they like but have a very difficult time sticking to things that aren't fun. Hyperactivity may include fidgeting and squirming, running, or climbing when inappropriate. Impulsivity may manifest as blurting out the answer before the question is finished, inability to wait one's turn, or interrupting frequently. ADHD can be primarily inattention, primary hyperactivity/impulsivity, or a combination of both. Left untreated, it is associated with lower academic performance, psychiatric conditions, and poor relationships with families and friends.

ADHD can be diagnosed by a pediatrician, psychologist, or psychiatrist. It is not necessary to get a neuropsychological evaluation to diagnose ADHD, but this can be very helpful to identify other learning or psychiatric issues. The healthcare professional will want to observe the child and talk to the parents and teachers about the child's behaviors. They will want to rule out other causes for the behavior such as depression, anxiety, and autism spectrum disorder.

Once a diagnosis of ADHD has been made, there are several treatment options. For preschoolers, the first line therapy is Parent Training in Behavior Management (PTBM). PTBM encourages consistently rewarding positive behaviors and ignoring or redirecting negative behaviors. When behavioral interventions do not provide significant improvement, consideration may be given to the use of the medication methylphenidate in 4- to 5-year-olds.

For school-aged children, a combination of behavioral interventions, educational accommodations, and medication has been shown to be most effective. Behavioral interventions include both PTBM and behavioral classroom intervention such as a reward system and daily report card. Educational accommodations should be detailed in an IEP or 504 Plan (see Question 74) and may include, for example, seating the student away from distractions and close to the teacher, frequent breaks, dividing long assignments into smaller parts, or extended time on assignments.

Medications can be very effective in treating ADHD. There is the strongest evidence to support the use of stimulants for ADHD. This may seem counterintuitive, but stimulants increase the amount of certain chemicals in the brain, dopamine and norepinephrine, that are needed for attention and motivation. Common stimulants include methylphenidate, dextroamphetamine, and dexmethylphenidate. Side effects from stimulants include loss of appetite, difficulty sleeping (if the dose is too high or the child metabolizes the drug slowly), irritability, headaches, and, rarely, tics. Stimulants can rarely cause abnormalities with heart rhythm. For those who don't tolerate stimulants, there are nonstimulant options, which include atomoxetine, guanfacine, and clonidine. These medications have different side effects. The good news is that ADHD is a treatable disorder often with a combination of behavioral therapy and medication.

Vicky's Comment:

My son showed signs of impulsivity, rigidity, and oppositional behavior, so we worked with a psychiatrist and a counselor and tried different medications to address these issues. Ultimately, we found a combination of two medications that together worked well for him; one addressed depression and anxiety and the other, ADHD. The combination of the two drugs worked on stabilizing his overall mood and behavior. It takes a little time to get the right medications in the right dosage.

80. How does one prepare a child with muscular dystrophy for college?

College may take the form of a public or private college where the student lives on or off campus versus online college where the student lives at home. College is a place to learn to think critically and develop deep knowledge. It is also a place to develop social skills, lasting friendships, and independence. Those with postsecondary education are more likely to get a job and have a higher salary. For all of these reasons, a child with MD should consider attending college. However, the process of preparing for college for a child with MD may take more resource navigation and planning than for those without MD.

Regardless of postsecondary education goals, transition planning is relevant to every child with MD. Transition planning should begin when the student is 13 or 14 years old. A child with MD will transition his or her health care, education, and potentially living environment all about the same time, around the age of adulthood. A detailed transition plan is thus necessary to prepare for this complex adjustment. There are planners such as the Transition Toolkit for DMD that can help assess the student's readiness for transition, track progress toward goals, and provide a guide to recording key pieces of medical and educational information about the transition process.[1]

During the early years of high school, the student should work on developing the skills that he or she will need to be successful in college. He or she will need to learn time management, organization skills, study skills, test-taking strategies, and stress management. The student should be encouraged to become involved in school or community-based activities. He or she should set goals and work toward achieving them. Along with his or her family and IEP team, the student should identify the educational, social, and physical supports that he or she needs to attain these goals. One aspect of identifying supports is fully exploring assistive technology.

At the beginning of high school, the student should be participating in his or her IEP meeting. Soon thereafter, the student should transition into leading the IEP meeting. This will reinforce the habit of advocating for oneself. In college, parents will no longer be advocating for the student who will be considered an adult and expected to make his or her own decisions.

This gradual transfer of responsibilities should be continued at home. The student should develop independent living skills. This can take the form of making decisions regarding care, performing household chores, driving, and/or managing money.

Teachers, parents, and healthcare professionals should discuss with the student future careers and aspirations. The student may be able to identify careers he or she would want to pursue and explore opportunities in that field with volunteer work or part-time jobs.

Later in high school, the student should visit several college campuses. In addition to assessing the location, size, fields of study, and atmosphere, the student will want to fully evaluate the support services. He or she should meet with the disability support services offices. It can be invaluable to speak to current college students or alumni with and without disabilities for their perspectives.

Not every child with MD desires a college education. However, students with MD should feel confident that they can attend if this is their goal. Many colleges are easily accessible with a wealth of support services (see https://www.collegexpress.com/lists/list/colleges-with-a-physically-disabled-friendly-environment/403/)

Tayjus' Comment:

It is important to realize that the transition to college is a major transition for all students, with or without MD. Everyone is likely struggling with some aspects of the transition, so parents or individuals with MD should not feel alone. Assuming that the students are interested in college and can handle the rigors, it is crucial that the individuals begin developing the confidence to advocate for themselves. When you have a disability, you may need to be able to speak up and advocate for yourself more than others. Parents should encourage the child to do things even as simple as ordering pizza and start to learn some independent living skills. Each person reaches these milestones at different points, so it may take longer for some. If possible, individuals should also start getting used to personal care assistants sooner rather than later so that they are prepared to manage their own care in college. If an individual does not feel ready to live away at school, they can also consider commuting. They should start talking to disability support services offices even while applying to understand what accommodations they might be able to receive. I also found it very helpful to see how others with MD were managing at college! That helped me realize that I too could live away from home and manage my care.

Reference

1. Trout CJ, et al. A transition toolkit for Duchenne muscular dystrophy. *Pediatrics* 2018;142(Suppl 2):S110–S117.

PART THIRTEEN

Work and Muscular Dystrophy

When and what should I share with my employer?

What are reasonable accommodations that a workplace should make?

Should I keep working?

More . . .

81. When and what should I share with my employer?

In general, you should disclose your disability when it is preventing you from competing for a job, performing a job, or gaining access to a benefit of employment. It is best to disclose your disability and request accommodations before your job performance suffers, as employers do not have to revoke any punitive actions that occurred before they were informed about your disability.

You do not need to disclose your diagnosis, but you do have to disclose that you have a disability and how it is affecting your job performance in order to receive accommodations. This may take the form of a statement such as, "Because of my disability, I am having trouble with X job duty." The employer may require medical documentation that you have an ADA disability and need accommodations. This can take the form of a letter from your doctor. You can instruct your doctor on how much information (e.g., your diagnosis) you want to disclose. Your employer does not have the right to request your medical records.

Your employer must keep information that you share with him/her confidential. For example, coworkers who may need to do something differently as a result of an accommodation may be told of the change required but not the reason why the change was made. Information on your disability and accommodations should never go in a personnel file.

When and what you share with your employer will be determined in part by your comfort level with the relationship. Some people feel that it is helpful to share early on and work with their employer as a team to establish accommodations. Others may want to share the bare minimum needed to understand their job performance. The ADA ensures that your employer cannot discriminate against you once you disclose.

82. What are reasonable accommodations that a workplace should make?

The ADA requires that employers make reasonable accommodations to those with disabilities so that they (1) have equal opportunity in the hiring process; (2) are able to perform their essential job functions; and (3) can enjoy equal benefits and privileges of employment. Employers who have 15 or more employees are required to provide reasonable accommodations, as are some state and local government employers.

A **reasonable accommodation** enables an individual with a disability to have an equal opportunity to get a job and to successfully perform the essential functions of that job. Such accommodations vary depending on the job duties of the employee, the environment, and employee's disability. Reasonable accommodations are ones that do not create undue hardship for the employer. Undue hardship includes accommodations that are very costly, extensive, or disruptive, or those that would fundamentally alter the nature or operation of the business. Unfortunately, this still leaves significant room for interpretation.

Reasonable accommodation
Modifications to a job or work environment an employer can make to enable an employee with a disability to perform essential functions of a job.

Here is a list of some reasonable accommodations that have been made by employers for those with MD:

- Providing reserved parking close to the entrance
- Installing a ramp
- Installing automatic door openers

- Modifying the layout of the workspace (e.g., moving workspace closer to bathroom, equipment, break room)
- Modifying a restroom
- Providing ergonomic equipment
- Providing telephone headset
- Providing speech recognition software
- Providing alternative keyboard, mouse
- Allowing a flexible work schedule
- Allowing periodic rest breaks
- Allowing longer bathroom breaks
- Allowing employee's personal care attendant
- Allowing employee's service animal
- Restructuring job duties

A couple of very helpful accommodations that may or may not be reasonable depending on the job and business include reassignment and work from home. If you can no longer perform your current job (for instance, one that involves travel) but could perform the functions of another job at the same company (for instance, a desk job), you may request reassignment. The employer does not have to create a new position or terminate or transfer other employees to reassign you. You must have the qualifications to perform the essential job duties of this new assignment.

Getting ready for work, commuting, navigating the workspace, and using the work bathrooms are all fatiguing and at times dangerous for those with MD. Working at home saves much-needed energy, is much more comfortable, and may be safer for those with difficulties ambulating or those needing daytime respiratory support. Many companies allow telecommuting and work remotely. Not all individuals function well in this setting however and before embarking on this transition there is a need for self-reflection on whether or not home is a good work environment for you.

To request accommodations at work, you must first disclose your disability (see Question 80). You are not required to submit your request in writing, but it is recommended that you do so that you have documentation in case there is any future dispute about your job performance or requested accommodation. As your needs change over time, you can request additional accommodations. Your employer must consider each request for reasonable accommodations on a case-by-case basis. You may need to provide some creative solutions to your work problems. And as in all aspects of life with MD, you will need to be a strong self-advocate.

Tayjus' Comment:

Under the ADA, employers are required to make accommodations for people with disabilities, but it does not mean that all employers will do a good job at accommodating those with disabilities. Many employers still have all sorts of misconceptions about people with disabilities and so the best option is to work for a large corporation or in the government where they are more likely to properly comply with the ADA. In many cases, these large companies already have things like ramps in places, but many other things are likely bigger fights. Much of this likely depends on if the company has ever hired people with similar needs. My employer has hired so many individuals with MD and other individuals with disabilities that they go above and beyond. They have a disability accommodations team and provide personal care assistants at work, accessible transportation to go from building to building, flexible work schedules, and will work to ensure you have what you need. It would be ideal if all companies could operate like this.

Lilleen's Comment:

I know that when I was working, I didn't want anyone, including my employer, to know that I had MD. That worked fine while I was young—in my 20s—because my challenges didn't interfere with my job. There was no need to ask for any special accommodations. However, as my FSHD progressed, I found it more and more difficult to continue to work. This was especially true if the weather was bad or the sidewalks and/or parking lots were slick. Most states have agencies to work with or even retrain people who become disabled. Additionally, they can mediate or work with you and your company. I strongly suggest that you become familiar with what is available in your state, as they all are different. Keep in mind that your challenge is progressive! Don't wait until you can no longer work or can't do a certain task. Be proactive.

83. Should I keep working?

Whether or not to keep working with a progressive MD is a difficult decision. Increasing weakness may make the physical demands of the job very difficult or impossible. The amount of energy that a job requires and the transportation to and from work may cause overwhelming fatigue with no remaining energy for life outside of work.

However, there are multiple benefits to continued employment that should be considered and may encourage you to seek accommodations that could make your job feasible. The obvious benefit is financial. Most full-time jobs pay substantially more than disability benefits. Employment benefits such as private health and dental insurance, contributions to 401(k)/403(b) plans or pensions, life insurance, etc., can be a significant incentive to stay. To receive the maximum retirement benefits from the Social Security Administration you need to contribute for a minimum of 10 years, although further contributions will not necessarily increase your monthly allowance.

There are often major social benefits to continued working. In your job you interact with a wealth of people including potentially peers, supervisors, staff, clients, etc. These social interactions boost physical and mental health. One of the risks of unemployment is social isolation. This is particularly true of those with MD who have challenges ambulating and are less likely to go out of the house. Social isolation is linked with depression, anxiety, and poor overall health outcomes.

Working provides opportunities to learn, develop skills, and think creatively. These mental benefits can be extremely rewarding and contribute to cognitive acuity. Early retirement has been linked to increased rates of dementia.

Many people derive a sense of identity and life purpose through meaningful work. Contributing to something larger than oneself gives motivation to get up out of bed each morning. This can be difficult to replace outside of work.

These are issues to consider when you are contemplating leaving the workforce. Before you leave, explore workplace accommodations (see Question 81) and consider shifting career paths to a job that is less physically demanding or one that would allow you to work from home. However, if you find that you cannot continue to work, map out a plan to try to replace some of the benefits of work with other activities. This may take the form of a part-time job, volunteering, or other community activity.

Tayjus' Comment:

This is always a huge question for people with MD. I think most of my friends with MD would all agree that they want to be independent, productive, social, and have some sort of life purpose. However, for most of my friends, the challenge is that we need either family or, more ideally, personal care assistants to help us with our activities of daily living. I need help from the time I wake up to the time I go to bed. Employment thus creates several logistical challenges. Furthermore, there is a major challenge of being able to afford personal care assistants. This is a huge expense well above the range that most people can afford. Thus, many people with MD must be on their state's Medicaid program as Medicaid will fund personal care assistants. But in order to receive Medicaid benefits, an individual has all sorts of asset and income limits. In a sense, many people with MD are disincentivized from working because they need the personal care benefits more than anything. It is often stressful to have to deal with Medicaid and personal care assistants, but it is worth it if you want to be employed and be independent. A lot of reform is still necessary.

Lilleen's Comment:

Unfortunately, for too many, the question becomes, can I afford to quit? My recommendation to you is that if you are currently employed, you should save as much money as you can. Live well below your means so that if and/or when the day comes that you can't work or don't want to continue working, you will have options. When I reached the point that I found going in to work to be too challenging, I decided to become self-employed. I found something I loved where I could work from home. Many more opportunities are available to work from home today than were available in years past.

84. What are disability benefits?

The Social Security Administration (SSA) has two programs that provide benefits for those with disabilities: Social Security Disability Insurance (SSDI) and Supplemental Security Income (SSI) programs. SSA defines disability as being unable to be gainfully employed due to a mental or physical ailment that is expected to cause death or that has lasted or is expected to last for at least 12 months. MD would fall under the covered entity of a neurological disorder. Disability may be demonstrated by poor motor function in two extremities with "extreme limitation" in ability to stand up from a seated position, balance while standing or walking, or use of the arms. Alternatively, disability may be demonstrated by a "marked limitation" in physical functioning and understanding, remembering, or applying information; interacting with others; concentrating, persisting, or maintaining pace or adapting or managing oneself. The Social Security website (https://www.ssa.gov/disability) provides examples of limitations in function that would be required for determination of disability.

SSDI is a benefit provided to disabled individuals who are "insured" by means of having worked and paid Social Security taxes (usually for at least 10 years). An adult child of an insured person may also receive benefits if his or her disability began before age 22. A spouse and minor children of a disabled individual eligible for SSDI may also receive benefits. Myotonic has prepared an excellent toolkit to help you through the application process: https://www.myotonic.org/sites/default/files /pages/files/Myotonic-MySSA-Toolkit-2019.pdf.

SSI is a benefit provided to disabled individuals of any age and also older adults age 65 and older who have limited income. SSA considers the income and re-sources of the parents when determining if a child will receive benefits. The amount of SSI benefit varies from state to state but is generally lower than SSDI benefits. In most states, individuals with SSI will automatically qualify for Medicaid.

Many individuals with MD have their first application for disability denied. With the assistance of your neurolo-gist and lawyer, you may need to resubmit the application. Because of this, you should plan financially for several months if not a couple years after your initial applica-tion is submitted and before receiving disability benefits. You may be able to avoid a denial by making sure that you have all the proper medical documentation. Ask your neurologist to read the SSA's qualifications for disability and carefully document your diagnosis, exam, functional capabilities, and supporting tests. A disability lawyer or advocate may not always be necessary but can steer you through the process and avoid costly denials and delays.

85. What is the Family and Medical Leave Act?

The Family and Medical Leave Act (FMLA) is a United States labor law that provides employees with job protection and unpaid leave for certain medical and family reasons. FMLA guarantees up to 12 weeks of unpaid leave during any 12-month period to care for the employee's spouse, child, or parent with a serious medical condition or for a serious health condition that makes the employee unable to perform the essential functions of his or her job. There are also provisions for the birth or adoption of a child and for family members of service members.

To be eligible for FMLA, an employee must have worked for the employer for at least 12 months, have worked at least 1250 hours over the past 12 months, and work for an employer with at least fifty employees. Some states allow for additional family and medical leave for employees and several states have thresholds lower than 50 employees, so it is worth checking your state's FMLA laws.

Although FMLA guarantees unpaid leave, you may be able to use paid leave that you have accrued on the job such as vacation days and sick days to receive pay during your leave. Some employers may require you to use up any paid leave that you have prior to taking leave under FMLA.

FMLA guarantees that you can return to your position or a position with equivalent pay, benefits, and responsibility. It also guarantees that you are afforded the same benefits while you are on leave.

You may be asked to provide a letter from your or your family member's doctor to your employer. However, you are not required to provide medical records.

One of the great benefits of FMLA is that the leave can be intermittent. Therefore, going to regular PT sessions or participating in a clinical trial for example would qualify for eligible leave under FMLA, in addition to continuous leave, such as hospitalization.

86. How do I get personal care attendant support?

Being independent, whether you are working, going to school, or staying at home, often depends on what kind of help you can get for ADLs. A personal care attendant or assistant (PCA) is an integral member of your team. A PCA can assist with getting in and out of bed, dressing, bathing, toileting, transfers, laundry, cooking, and light housework, and for more complex needs, care for a tracheostomy or G-tube. A PCA can be a family member, student, agency employee, certified nursing assistant, or registered nurse depending on your needs. You may choose to have multiple PCAs who work in shifts or a live-in PCA.

There are many approaches to finding a PCA. You could advertise independently, for example on roommate forums or at nursing and physical therapy schools. If you are in college, you might find a fellow student interested in working with you through campus publications or bulletin boards. Employment agencies keep lists of people looking for employment and can connect you to a PCA. If you hire independently, you will be responsible for paying the PCA directly and for the PCA's taxes and liability insurance. Unless you make arrangements with another PCA or family member, you will not have backup if the PCA is unable to come to work.

Alternatively, you could use a home health agency to supply PCAs. In this case, you may have less say in who is working for you. However, the agency will be responsible for doing a background check, paying the PCA (and billing you for services), and for taxes and insurance. They will likely provide backup if the PCA is unable to come to work.

In selecting a PCA or a home health agency, you will want to conduct an interview and check references. During an interview, you should describe in detail your day, your needs, and what the responsibilities will be of the PCA as well as the schedule. You should ask questions such as the PCA's experience, habits, reasons for wanting to be a PCA, and how he or she would handle an emergency. If hiring from a home health agency, you will want to know, for example, if they have any experience working with people with similar needs, what qualifications their PCAs have, whether you can be involved in selecting the specific PCA who will be working with you, what are their emergency procedures, and what are the procedures if you are unhappy with their PCA. Experience is certainly a plus, but perhaps the most important aspects to discern from an interview are compatibility, empathy, and good communication skills.

PCAs are expensive. Medicare does not cover non-medical PCAs. Private insurance usually does not either. Medicaid will cover PCAs, but there are qualifying limits to income and assets. In some states, Medicaid and state-funded programs will provide for a family member to act as a PCA.

While working with a PCA you should strive to maintain a friendly but professional relationship. It is helpful to set clear boundaries. You should feel comfortable asking your PCA to do the things that you have outlined in the job description. Your ability to communicate well and be a good self-advocate will be important for a successful relationship. The job pays minimally, and your show of appreciation for the PCA's efforts will go a long way.

Tayjus' Comment:

PCAs are critical to being independent when you have MD and need help with ADLs. PCAs have made it possible for me to attend a college and now have a job far from home. During my first year of college, my parents and I decided we should go through a home health agency for PCAs because it was all new to us. We felt that the agency would remove the stresses of having to find a PCA and concerns about needing a backup PCA. In my experience, I actually do not think that using a home health agency for PCAs is the best option. I found that the PCAs provided through the agency were more unprofessional and simply did not understand the idea of independent living. Most home health agency PCAs are used to seniors and as a result are simply not the right fit for active younger individuals. After my first year and mediocre experience with a home health agency, I decided to go about recruiting and hiring PCAs on my own, something I observed many others with MD doing. I have found that word of mouth has been the best way because these PCAs have already been screened and have likely already done very similar tasks. I have also used Care.com and Craigslist. When I use these services, I always include a survey to essentially screen out candidates before I reach out to them for interviews. I personally do not care if the PCA has any previous background as I would rather train them to do things exactly the way that I want them to. It is important to remember that the PCA works for you and should do things the way you want them to. You will inevitably be in situations where you need to advocate for yourself and will need to address issues with the PCAs. You may need to correct them, set boundaries, or even confront them about being late for example. It is not fun, but it prepares you for the real world and having to manage people. PCAs are not paid much for all they do, and it is important to look past some of the negatives. It can be hard to find good PCAs, so it is important to focus on their positives and learn to ignore certain things.

Vicky's Comment:

Having a PCA over the past three years has been both the biggest blessing as well as one of the most challenging aspects of living with DMD. Qualifications, experience, and references are all extremely valuable but the most important thing, in our experience, has been personality and compatibility. The job requires the caregiver to help with many personal needs such as toileting, dressing, feeding, etc. This is a hard situation for a young man to be in as it is, so making sure there is a level of trust, respect, and professionalism is crucial. We had a bad experience with a caregiver once, who left my son on the toilet to "teach him a lesson" about patience. It was very poor judgment to leave my son in a vulnerable position and to discipline with a basic need. Needless to say, this person was let go, and every interview with a caregiver, thereafter, involved questions about disciplining and outlining what steps to take when my son was not behaving appropriately. It was an important lesson for all of us.

PART FOURTEEN

Play and Muscular Dystrophy

What are adaptive sports?

What options are there for a computer mouse or controller?

What are appropriate limits for video games and online socialization?

More . . .

87. What are adaptive sports?

Adaptive sports or parasports includes a wide range of sports or recreational activities that have been modified for those with disabilities. Adaptive sports provide many benefits including muscle toning, cardiovascular conditioning, social interactions, and fun. Team sports teach teamwork and leadership. There are many sports those with MD can enjoy with a few adaptations. Adaptive sports help realize an individual's potential.

There are many different types of adaptive sports. Here are a few that my patients have participated in.

- **Hippotherapy** or therapeutic horseback riding provides excellent exercise to the legs and core musculature and emotional benefits from working with animals (https://americanhippotherapy association.org/).
- **Adaptive swimming** provides excellent exercise to muscles of the arms, legs, and core, improves flexibility, and provides cardiovascular conditioning (https://www.disabledsportsusa.org/sport /swimming/).
- **Power soccer** is a sport for those using a wheelchair. A guard can be attached to the front of the wheelchair for "kicking" the ball. There are many power soccer leagues for children and adults throughout the country, which can be quite competitive (https://www.powersoccerusa.org).
- **Wheelchair tennis** is a similarly rewarding and competitive sport for those with preserved arm function, with leagues and tournaments throughout the country (https://www.usta.com).
- **Adaptive skiing** is a sport open to people of all levels of disability. For standing individuals,

four-track skiing includes two outriggers, which are metal crutches with ski tips at the ends. Others can sit in a bucket attached to one or two skis (https://www.disabledsportsusa.org/sport /downhill-skiing/).

- **Sailing** in specially rigged boats is also available to people at all levels of disability (see **Figure 12**). For racing, sailors are classified by their degree of disability (https://www.ussailing.org/education/adult /adaptive-sailing/).

Many of these sports, including horseback riding, swimming, skiing, and sailing, provide individuals with an incredible sense of freedom. Beyond the health benefits, MD athletes report increased self-confidence, empowerment, and independence that extend to other aspects of life.

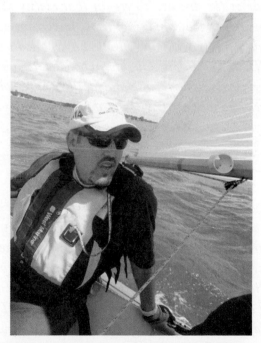

Figure 12 An individual with DM1 enjoying adaptive sailing.

Tayjus' Comment:

As a kid, I did take part in a couple adaptive sports. I remember going to hippotherapy as a young kid, and I really enjoyed it. It was something I always remember fondly. I also briefly was on a baseball team for kids with special needs. From around age 7 to 18, I did go to an adaptive swimming program at our local YWCA. This is something I also really enjoyed, and I always felt good when I went swimming. I would usually hold onto a noodle and the person with me would guide me. I also have many MD friends who compete in power soccer, which they really enjoy.

Lilleen's Comment:

Adaptive skiing was so much fun, and challenging. It gave me back something that I thought I had lost the ability to do because of the disease. To regain that ability through a few adaptations was amazing. Most important was now I could do something fun with my son who too is affected by FSHD, and with my daughter who loves to snowboard. Adaptive sports allows friends and family who are physically challenged and who are physically abled to do things together that maybe they once thought was lost.

Colin's Comment:

It is important for all of us to find something we are passionate about in our lives. Something that gets us out of bed in the morning, something that we find rewarding, fulfilling, and satisfying. Sailing is my passion, but after being diagnosed with MD, I thought it was one more physical activity that I could no longer do. Then I discovered adaptive sailing and got back out on the water. It was amazing, the change it made in my life. I started to feel things I hadn't experienced in a long time—feelings like *hope, empowerment, and freedom. Becoming involved in adaptive sailing is one of the best decisions I ever made. Being around other sailors with MD (and other disabilities) made me realize that I could be a sailor first and disabled second. Most importantly because of the technology that has been and is being developed to allow disabled people to sail, I should be able to sail for as much of my future as I want to regardless of the progression of my MD.*

88. What options are there for a computer mouse or controller?

If use of a standard mouse becomes difficult, there are multiple options that are available to maintain independence with computer access. The first strategy may be to simply adjust the mouse speed within the controls of the computer. Alternative mouse options are also available and vary greatly in complexity and cost. Selecting the right mouse for you depends upon combining the most accurate motor control with the least energy expenditure.

Currently, several alternative mouse options include:

- Different size, style, and ergonomic mice
- Track pads (some of which can be programmable for limited range of motion)
- Track ball (handheld finger track ball mouse can be held in the palm of the hand with single thumb or finger movement for activation)
- Keyboard key pad
- Phone app for mouse control
- Joystick, free standing with varying degrees of programmability
- Wheelchair driving controls—many current wheelchair joysticks and alternative driving

controls can also be used for mouse control via Bluetooth

- Switch access via scanning or radar mouse
- Head pointing
- Voice control
- Eye gaze

Technology is constantly changing and alternative methods for controlling your mouse, computer, and tablet are also continuing to evolve, with increasing options also built into the computer or tablet. Although there are many options commercially available, an evaluation with an occupational therapist or assistive technology professional may help you determine the most effective option for mouse control. The purchase of equipment to access a computer or tablet is not covered by insurance, so it may be prudent to trial the equipment before purchase.

Vicky's Comment:

It became very apparent one day when my son was unable to use the mouse for our main desk top computer. We were using a Mac and visited the Apple store the next day and the salesperson recommended a great ergonomically designed track pad that worked perfectly for my son. On his phone and iPad, he also used apps like swipe, to enable him to drag his fingers along a few letters that the device then recognized as the word. This was a great help and came at just the right time for him.

89. What are appropriate limits for video games and online socialization?

Media in the form of streaming television, interactive video games, and social media play a prominent role in the lives of many with MD. It can be entertaining, educational, social, and creative. Many of the interactive games provide rich worlds in which an individual with MD does not have a disability. They also provide a link to a wide world of online friendships when MD can be otherwise socially isolating.

However, media can also replace in-person socialization, family time, schoolwork, physical activity, enjoyment reading, and sleep. Time spent online becomes a problem if it leads to loss of interest in other activities, withdrawal, or deception. For this reason, many families look for suggestions on media time limits.

The American Academy of Pediatrics (AAP) recommends that for those under 6 years of age, a limit be set to 1 hour of high-quality educational programming. For older ages, the amount of time is dependent on the specific child and family. American Academy of Pediatrics suggests making a Family Media Use Plan (www.HealthyChildren.org/MediaUsePlan) to explore time commitments to other activities and set consistent limits to screen time. It is recommended that there are screen-free zones such as the dinner table and device curfews. Media devices should not be present in the bedroom and should be turned off 1 hour before bedtime to ensure restful sleep.

As important to quantity of screen time is quality. Parents should select and view media with children identifying high-quality, age-appropriate, and safe sites. They should discuss cyberbullying, sexting, online predators, personal privacy, and safety. They should also remind the child surfing the internet that not everything they read about MD is accurate or relevant to his or her disease.

Video games and online socialization can provide a creative and social outlet for those with MD. The trick is to maintain balance ensuring enough sleep, in person social time, schoolwork, etc. The content of screen time and degree to which screen time substitutes for other healthy activities are aspects that every family should monitor in addition to total screen time.

Vicky's Comment:

This is a topic of great interest and concern to both MD and nonMD families. My son is 17 and we still have to monitor his screen time. It is always an easier option to escape into the world of games and fantasy. However, a growing concern of this generation is that people and experiences are what bring joy and happiness to life, not isolated imaginary play. We make an effort to have game night, where we play various board games and family meetings where we all share what's happening in our lives; proud moments and struggles. We love to travel, discuss politics, and cook together. My son is a real foodie and his job is to find recipes, source the ingredients, read directions, and keep time of each stage of preparation. Finally, he's the official taste tester before a dish is brought to the table. My son is also very fond of sporting events and concerts, so we try to do an event of his choice three or four times a year.

90. What are some tips for airplane travel?

Travel can be exciting and fulfilling. It can also cause stress if you have impaired mobility. Prior planning for airplane travel is necessary to reduce this stress and ensure everything goes well.

Know your passenger rights as set forth by the U.S. Department of Transportation and carry a copy of these rights with you: https://www.transportation.gov/air consumer/fly-rights. Call your airline carrier well in advance of your trip and describe your needs. Many airlines also have a place to request special assistance when making your booking.

You will want to preboard the airplane to give yourself additional time to get situated. You might tell the gate agent about how many minutes it will take you to get situated if you know so that you do not feel pressured to hurry with other passengers behind you. If you are ambulatory, you might consider the use of a cane (even if you don't normally use one) as a visual aid to others that you need time and should not be jostled. If you use a wheelchair, ask to ride your wheelchair to the entrance of the plane and then transfer to an onboard wheelchair for the transfer to your seat. There is storage inside the cabin for a collapsible manual wheelchair. A motorized wheelchair will need to go in cargo. You will want to ask someone to remove all the loose pieces of your wheelchair such as your footrests and pack these so that they don't become lost in the flight. Check with the airline beforehand that your battery is of the type that is allowed on the plane. Bring a small bag of tools to perform minor repairs in case the airline damages the wheelchair. Damage to wheelchairs is so common that many fliers prefer to use an old wheelchair when they travel and leave their favorite one at home. However, if your wheelchair is damaged, the airline is responsible for replacement or repairs and for providing you a loaner in the interim.

Remember that your medical equipment (including BIPAP, CPAP, cane, etc.) does not count as carry-on luggage. You can't be certain that there will be a power outlet available, so bring battery-operated ventilator support if you need it. Ask that the onboard wheelchair remain on the plane for the duration of the flight to assist you with using the bathrooms.

For domestic flights, the bathrooms are quite small and are not large enough to fit the onboard wheelchair and another person to help with transfers. There are regulations for two-aisle planes that include larger bathrooms, which are accessible, but these also may be too small. If you are a male, you might consider the use of a condom catheter, which is attached to a bag for urine that is strapped around the leg. This allows you to urinate freely without having to transfer in a small bathroom. Unfortunately, for a woman there is not a similar contraption for urination, but the use of a diaper, although not sexy, may be more practical than trying to use the airplane toilet.

Accessible travel is becoming more and more available throughout the world. It requires advanced planning and self-advocacy. With that, the rewards are great.

Tayjus' Comment:

When I fly, I take my chair all the way up to the door of the plane and then transfer into the aisle chair. To transfer, I use a sling called the "comfort carrier," which requires two people to grab the handles. This took some getting used to, but it has made flying easier. In the past, when my chair had removable footrests, I would remove them. My rule of thumb is to remove anything that could come off. I don't usually carry a lot of wheelchair tools other than perhaps a multitool. I also always create signage for the chair explaining how to turn on the chair, put it into manual mode, recline the chair if needed to fit in the hold, and I emphasize that the chair is my legs and to handle with care. I also call ahead to ensure that they know my needs. Upon arriving at the gate, I go to the gate agent and request that they send up the ground supervisor so I can explain how my chair operates. Upon arrival, if there is any damage to the chair, it is best to go complain right away so that the airline can begin the process to have things repaired.

Vicky's Comment:

From our experience, airlines are usually very helpful in navigating wheelchair friendly procedures that include early boarding and the use of an aisle chair provided by the airline. We travel with an electric scooter that can be dismantled into three parts, and we are able to drive it up to the gate and transfer to their aisle chair. The scooter is then available at the gate on the other end, as a baby stroller would be. Planning and informing the airline in advance is always beneficial.

Colin's Comment:

As a veteran flier of multiple cross-country flights, I have learned many lessons about air travel with a disability like MD. Unfortunately, even with prior planning, there is ample opportunity for things to go wrong. Even though I am ambulatory, I use a wheelchair when I fly. Walking long distances and standing in the airport are difficult. When I book my flights, I request that a wheelchair be waiting at my destination. It's problematic if the wheelchair isn't there when the plane reaches the gate. I've had to wait on the plane until the mass exodus of passengers getting off is over. This is not to say that I have encountered problems on every flight, but it illustrates that no matter how much you plan in advance, complications do occur. I find the best way to handle this is to arrive at the airport early and always have a travel companion. I think that the two most important things to make air travel with MD safe and comfortable are tolerance and a sense of humor.

PART FIFTEEN

Sexual Health Issues

What about dating and sex?

What if I want to get pregnant?

91. *What about dating and sex?*

Individuals with MD have sexual and emotional needs just like everyone else. While there is person to person variability influenced by biology, culture, and life experiences, most individuals with MD desire emotional and physical intimacy. They are certainly all deserving of love.

Within the general public, there is a common misconception that people with disabilities are not able to have sex. This may arise from portrayals of patients with spinal cord injuries, many of whom have lost sensation below a certain spinal cord level. However, this is not true of people with MD. Sensation is intact, and involuntary muscles important in sexual function are minimally if at all affected. There may be logistic challenges to sexual activities because of weakness and/or contractures. These challenges can often be overcome with some imagination, devices, and good partner communication. Some medications that individuals with MD may be prescribed, such as beta blockers or antidepressants, can reduce libido or sexual function. Discuss these concerns with your doctor, who may be able to recommend alternative medications or suggest other solutions.

A greater challenge for many individuals with MD is establishing a relationship. Finding a compatible partner and dating is hard enough when you don't have a serious medical condition. For some individuals with MD, difficulty with mobility may make it hard to get out and meet people. For others, the difficulty may be more with social interactions. These are significant challenges for which there is no easy solution. However, it may help to remember all that you can bring to a relationship. Others will value many of your unique qualities including resilience, determination, and humor that were forged through living with MD.

92. What if I want to get pregnant?

Having children is rewarding, and many young women with MD look forward to pregnancy and parenthood. With some exceptions, women with MD can have a healthy pregnancy and delivery. However, there are some risks to be aware of and some special planning that is needed to ensure that both mother and baby do well.

Before getting pregnant, please speak with your neurologist and genetics counselor to understand the risk of passing on MD to your child (see Question 11) and to understand your reproductive options. Your neurologist can also address your specific risks in regard to pregnancy, some of which are described in general terms below.

For those MDs that affect cardiac and pulmonary function, it is important to have these systems fully evaluated prior to pregnancy. Pregnancy puts increased demands on the heart. If you have an MD that affects the heart, it is possible that function may deteriorate during pregnancy. For this reason, your cardiologist may recommend against pregnancy if you have reduced heart function. An echocardiogram or cardiac MRI prior to pregnancy to assess function is recommended. Pregnancy also puts additional stress on the muscles of respiration. As the abdomen expands, it pushes on the diaphragm used for breathing. For those with limitations in their breathing, pulmonary function may further decline during pregnancy requiring ventilatory assistance. Pulmonary function testing prior to pregnancy is also recommended.

For most MDs, women do not have problems conceiving. The exception to this is DM1, which has higher rates of infertility. DM1 also has higher rates of miscarriages.[1]

Rapid weight gain and a changed center of gravity with pregnancy affect strength, balance, and walking ability. Many women with MD report a worsening of their weakness during pregnancy that did not return to baseline following delivery. Those with borderline ambulatory ability may need assistive devices during and potentially after pregnancy.

Due to potential complications with delivery, you will want to discuss your MD with your obstetrician so he or she is prepared. The first stage of labor, which requires the smooth muscle of the uterus to contract, is usually not problematic in MD, as smooth muscle is generally not affected. The exception to this is in DM, which may have difficulty progressing to the second stage of labor. In the second stage, uterine contractions are combined with voluntary contraction of abdominal muscles to push the baby out. Since abdominal muscles may be weakened in MD, there is an increased likelihood that interventions such as cesarean section or forceps delivery will be necessary. The third stage of labor, when the uterus contracts and expels the placenta, can again be a problem with DM. There is an increased rate of peripartum hemorrhage in DM (bleeding before, during, and after delivery).[1]

You should also have a preoperative evaluation with an anesthesiologist so that he or she is aware of your MD and potential complications. As discussed in Question 72, there are some precautions that should be taken with anesthesiology in MD, and pain medications may have greater or prolonged affects requiring more extensive monitoring.

With precautions and some exceptions, women with MD can become pregnant and safely deliver healthy babies. Although weakness may progress during pregnancy, the vast majority of women who have MD would choose to become pregnant again.[2]

Lilleen's Comment:

I'm not sure if being pregnant affected the progression of my FSHD or not. I was already experiencing some issues prior to becoming pregnant. What I would say is there are a wide variety of strains that affect the body during pregnancy. This would include things such as the extra weight your body must now carry, so watching my weight was very important. Since my stomach muscles were already weaker, I was placed on bed rest during the last trimester of both of my pregnancies. I also made sure I was followed by a specialist who dealt with high-risk pregnancies. Taking care of a baby afterward can also be a huge challenge depending on your body's weaknesses. Lifting, carrying, and bending over—all of these can also take a toll on the muscles. If you are considering having a child, you should first ask yourself, can I take care of this infant, can I afford to hire help if not, or do I have family support to help me? You can't control what happens to your body or the disease, but you can control some of the other factors. I don't have any regrets about having children.

References

1. Johnson NE, et al. The impact of pregnancy on myotonic dystrophy: a registry-based study. *Journal of Neuromuscular Diseases* 2015;2:447–452.

2. Ciafaloni E, et al. Pregnancy and birth outcomes in women with facioscapulohumeral muscular dystrophy. *Neurology* 2006;67: 1887–1889.

PART SIXTEEN

Assistive Equipment

Should I get a scooter or a wheelchair?

What features should I look for in a wheelchair?

What is a stander?

More . . .

93. Should I get a scooter or a wheelchair?

When first transitioning to a power mobility device, you may have questions about whether a power scooter or a power wheelchair better fits your needs. There are advantages and disadvantages to both and there are several factors to consider in making your choice with the help of your healthcare providers.

Power Scooters

A power scooter may be the first power mobility device utilized, but recommendation of a power scooter is dependent upon the individual's ability to sit without support, adequate upper extremity muscle strength to operate the tiller, the rate of muscle weakness progression, and the environment/s in which power mobility is needed. Advantages and disadvantages of a power scooter include:

- Advantages
  - Lighter weight
  - Foldable or can disassemble for transport
  - Seat can swivel on most models for transfers and table/countertop access
  - Seat can elevate on some models for ease of transfers
- Disadvantages
  - Limited ability to customize
  - Does not provide postural support if needed
  - Requires adequate upper extremity muscle strength to operate tiller
  - Large turning radius, limiting indoor maneuverability

- No power seating features are available
- Limited ability to handle outdoor terrain (uneven grassy areas, loose gravel, cobblestone, etc.)
- Reduced speed as compared to a power wheelchair (maximum speed is typically 4–5 mph)

Power scooters come in both 3-wheel and 4-wheel models. A 3-wheel power scooter is more maneuverable and typically recommended if the scooter is to be used primarily in the home, school, or work environments. A 4-wheel scooter is less maneuverable, but is more stable on outdoor surfaces. A 4-wheel scooter is more likely to be recommended if the scooter's primary use is in the community.

Although there are a multitude of lightweight or travel scooters on the market, as well as scooters designed with more all-terrain features; these are not generally covered by insurance. Many insurance carriers will only pay for a mobility device that can be used and is needed within the home environment. Even if the individual is still ambulating within his or her home, reduced balance and/or falls in the home may be medical justification for a power scooter.

Power Wheelchair

A dedicated power wheelchair is much more customizable than a power scooter and can provide greater postural support through use of a wide range of positioning components. A variety of power seat functions and driving controls are also available to specifically meet the individual needs of the wheelchair user. A power wheelchair is typically more maneuverable than a power scooter, but it is also heavier and typically requires use of an adapted vehicle for transport. Advantages and disadvantages of a power wheelchair include:

- Advantages
  - Can be highly customizable
  - Postural supports and driving methods can be changed or adapted as needed
  - Power seating options that are controllable by the wheelchair user are available, including tilt, recline, elevating leg rests, seat elevate, and standing
  - Smaller turning radius and more maneuverable within the home environment than a power scooter
  - Designed to handle outdoor terrain better than a power scooter
  - Operable at higher speeds; maximum is speed typically 6.0 to 6.5 mph, but higher speed packages may be available up to 8.5 mph
  - Larger batteries resulting in further driving distance per charge
- Disadvantages
  - Heavy
  - Most cannot fold or disassemble for transport and require an adapted vehicle (van with ramp or lift)

Although there are many lightweight/foldable power wheelchair options, as well as rugged, heavy-duty, all-terrain power chairs on the market, these are not generally covered by insurance. Many insurance carriers will only pay for a mobility device that can be used and is needed within the home environment. In order to qualify for a power wheelchair, documentation needs to be provided as to why other, less expensive devices (including canes, walkers, manual wheelchairs, and power scooters) cannot meet the client's mobility needs within their home environment. This documentation is provided by your neurologist, physical therapist, occupational therapist, and/or seating specialist.

Unless there is a change in diagnoses or significant change in medical condition, many insurance carriers will also only pay for a new mobility device every five years and only with documentation as to why the current power mobility system cannot be repaired or can no longer meet the medical needs of the client. Funding is usually covered before the five-year period for new seating components or postural supports due to growth, significant wear, or change in medical condition.

When selecting an appropriate mobility base, it is important to consider not only your current mobility needs, but also your anticipated needs over the next several years. Healthcare professionals who can help you with deciding between a power scooter or power wheelchair include your neurologist, physical therapist, and occupational therapist.

Lilleen's Comment:

The decision to get either a scooter or a wheelchair was one of the most difficult and emotional decisions that I've ever made. Transitioning to a scooter or wheelchair does not mean you necessarily have to stop walking; for some, it could be to conserve energy, while for others it could be to prevent falls. Whatever the reason, remember your safety should always be your first priority. My first scooter was big and bulky, and I absolutely hated it. I resisted using the scooter and would only use it if we were going somewhere that required a lot of walking. However, I was falling a lot more at home, and one day I found myself alone, with all the doors locked, and I could not get up. That's when I decided to transition to using the scooter when I was home alone. However, my resistance to using it full time was still very high; I felt using it was giving up. My doctor helped me to put things in perspective by telling me I wasn't giving up, I was preserving my energy. Finally, using my scooter full time, my whole world changed. Then, instead of being limited in where I went because of the physical demands, I was able to go and not worry about falling, wearing out my body, or being in so much pain that I couldn't move the next day. Whatever you decide to get, if you are using it to go places, you need to consider how it will be transported. Although many scooters are much more portable, they still require someone with strength to take them apart and lift them into the trunk of your car. Most wheelchairs require a mobility conversion van. Talk with others, both those who have a scooter and those who have a wheelchair. I would also recommend trying out several, maybe even renting one for the day. The most wonderful part about all of this is that it has returned my freedom to get out of my house!

94. What features should I look for in a wheelchair?

A wheelchair provides you with the ability to navigate the world. If you have lost the ability to safely ambulate, you may be spending a substantial portion of your day in your wheelchair. It is a big investment, costing as much as a nice car, and you will likely only get a new one every several years. For all these reasons, it is important that your wheelchair be specifically fitted for you with the features that help you successfully perform the activities that you want to do each day. Here are a few considerations:

Power Wheelchair Bases

Power wheelchair bases can be divided into 3 categories: rear wheel, mid wheel, and front wheel drive.

- *Rear wheel drive* is typically the least utilized, as it often has a larger turning radius. However, there are hybrid rear wheel drive chairs now available where the rear wheel has been brought further forward so that the turning radius is significantly reduced. Higher speed packages are more often available on the rear wheel drive chairs due to the greater stability/design of the base.

- *Mid wheel drive* has the smallest turning radius and is therefore most maneuverable in the home, school, and work environments. This style base is most frequently utilized unless power standing is necessary. Some mid wheel drive power wheelchairs offer power standing, but a full upright position cannot be achieved with this wheel configuration.

- *Front wheel drive* has a wider turning radius and is less maneuverable indoors but is able to handle more rugged outdoor terrain. A front wheel drive power wheelchair is required if power standing is necessary and a full upright standing position is desired.

Power Seating Features

In addition to selecting an appropriate power mobility base, determining the necessary power seating features will help narrow down the specific wheelchair that best meets your needs. Power seating features that are available include:

- *Power tilt* enables the wheelchair seat frame to tilt back while maintaining a constant seat-to-back angle. Power tilt is recommended for pressure relief and to minimize the risk of skin breakdown resulting from prolonged sitting. It is important for those individuals who are unable to perform and maintain a full weight shift or for those who have trunk and/or neck weakness. Power tilt also enables a position for rest and is important when fatigue may be a factor throughout the day.

- *Power recline* allows the back of the wheelchair to recline independently of the seat and opens the seat to back angle. Power recline is also helpful with pressure relief. It can be used fully or only in small increments to help and alleviate hip and back pain or strain and to stretch out tight hip flexors. Fully reclining the back can be useful for lower extremity dressing while in the wheelchair and partially reclining the back can be helpful when using a urinal or with catheter management from the wheelchair.

- *Power elevating leg rests* combined with power tilt can help to reduce **edema** (swelling) and improve circulation. If ordering the power recline feature, elevating leg rests are necessary to reduce strain on the lower back when reclining. Elevating leg rests can also be beneficial in stretching tight hamstrings and maintaining range of motion.

- *Power seat elevate* allows vertical adjustment of the seat height by the wheelchair user. Raising the seat height to transfer is critical for many individuals due to hip and knee weakness, which makes it impossible for them to stand from a standard seat height and transfer independently. Power elevation can also promote independence and/ or safety with lateral transfers by enabling a level transfer or a transfer from a higher to lower surface

Edema

Swelling of a body part, for example, in the legs of those sitting in a wheelchair.

that is gravity assisted. Power seat elevate can also facilitate greater participation in ADLs in the home, school, work, and community environments by extending the individual's arm reaching ability and increasing access to various height tables, desks, countertops, sinks, etc. Power seat elevation can reduce cervical strain and pain associated with always looking up from a seated position. It also provides psychosocial benefits of allowing the wheelchair user to be on the same level with peers and speaking eye-to-eye.

- *Power anterior tilt* allows forward tilting of the wheelchair while the seat remains at a fixed angle. This is also referred to as "active reach" and is available up to 30 degrees. A chest strap is required when any degree of trunk weakness is present, and both a chest strap and knee blocks are required for all clients depending on the degree of anterior tilt desired. This feature can help to promote independence or assistance with forward transfers. It can also increase the distance an individual can reach by shifting the center of gravity further forward over the wheelchair base and footrests, enabling the wheelchair user to get closer to countertops, sinks, desks, etc., that aren't cut out at the base for wheelchair access. Anterior tilt also shifts the individual's weight further forward over his or her feet and can provide a limited degree of modified leg weight bearing. It is not recommended for individuals with significant upper trunk and neck weakness.

- *Power standing* enables the wheelchair user to rise to a supported standing position from a seated position independently while remaining in the wheelchair. Many individuals who require standing for therapeutic reasons have been prescribed separate standers (see Question 95). However, use of a dedicated stander is often confined to once a day or less within a single environment and may require one or more care providers to transfer into the stander. With the power standing feature, an individual can assume a standing position independently from his or her wheelchair multiple times throughout the day and can drive the power chair in a standing position on level surfaces. See Question 95 for more information about the benefits of standing. However, it is important to be aware that power standing is not medically recommended for everyone. Standing may not be recommended in the presence of severe joint contractures, significant postural asymmetries, joint laxity, or decreased upper trunk and neck control. It is also important to note that power standing adds greater weight to the wheelchair, and often a larger base with greater turning radius is required.

Controls

Determining and selecting the most efficient way to control the power wheelchair and power seating features are also critical. Use of a joystick is the most standard method of driving. However, different style joysticks are available, and the location of the joystick can be altered if needed via an appropriate mount. Various joystick handles can be added for individuals with weak hand grip. Smaller and more sensitive joysticks that require significantly less pressure to operate are also available. Other types of hand controls such as touch pads and switches (microlight and/or infrared), as well as alternative driving methods including head control systems, eye gaze, and single switch scanning, may also be considered.

Postural Supports

In addition to the power base, power seating features, and drive/control method, the actual postural supports within a power wheelchair are typically customizable. During an evaluation for a power wheelchair, options for each of the following seating features should be discussed:

- Back support
- Lateral and anterior trunk support
- Seat cushion
- Arm support
- Leg support (pelvis, upper and lower leg, and foot)
- Headrest

Different supports may be needed depending on sitting balance, muscle weakness, range-of-motion limitations, skin integrity, orthopedic considerations, postural asymmetries, sitting tolerance (pain and/or fatigue), and functional activities performed in the wheelchair.

Although there are power add-on units for manual wheelchairs, as well as other lightweight or foldable power chairs on the market, they are less customizable, offer few if any power seating features, and offer limited driving control and seating options. These types of wheelchairs are typically not adaptable enough to meet an individual's needs when there is progressive muscle weakness or anticipation of change in medical condition.

When pursuing insurance coverage for a power wheelchair, the power base, power seating features, drive control features, and all seating/postural components need to be individually medically justified. Before ordering a power chair, various power mobility bases and seating features should be considered, demonstrated, and tried out by the individual. A seating specialist (often an occupational therapist or physical therapist) will work with you and your neurologist to identify your needs and help you select the features that will make you the most comfortable, promote the best health, and make you most successful in your activities.

Tayjus' Comment:

When you spend most of your day in a wheelchair, it is so important to have a chair that is comfortable, properly fitted, and that can do what you need. For me, the cushion has always been critical and the proper knee guides that help prevent my legs from splaying outward and my feet turning. I also use the tilt in space, recline, and the power footrest, which are crucial for relieving pressure during the day and being comfortable in general. The seat elevator is also great for reaching higher counters or in a social setting so that I can be eye level with others. I also prefer that the chair has a smaller profile so that it is easier to turn or fit into smaller spaces.

95. What is a stander?

A stander is a piece of equipment that supports the individual while he or she is standing. Use of a stander generally begins when the individual has limited walking or is nonambulatory. There are multiple benefits to maintaining standing with use of a stander. This includes maintenance of bone density, reduction of development of contractures, and digestive, respiratory, and cardiovascular benefits. It can be helpful to get off one's seat to prevent development of pain and pressure ulcers. Finally, there are psychological benefits to a stander in being able to meet people at eye level and see the world from a standing vantage point.

Standers come in different sizes for children and adults (see **Figure 13**). It is important to work with your physical therapist to find a stander that fits you appropriately. There are also different types of standers that your physical therapist may recommend: upright, prone (tilted forward), and supine (tilted backward). If you have low bone density, a prone or supine stander may be recommended to prevent fractures while in the stander. Mobile standers allow you to move about while

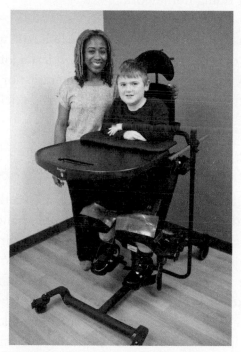

Figure 13 This young man with DMD is demonstrating the use of a stander alongside his physical therapist. Notice the large tray that can be used for homework, meals, or video games.

in a standing position. Wheelchairs with a standing feature (see Question 94) reduce the number of transfers required and improve functional reach and access to enable participation in activities such as grooming, cooking, toileting, reaching medications, etc., and provide mobility.

How much time you spend in your stander each day varies with the individual, presence of contractures, and comfort level. In general, 1 hour of standing a day is a good goal. This does not need to occur all at one time and can be broken up into smaller segments. Standing can occur when playing video games, watching a movie, eating, or doing homework.

Many insurance companies and Medicare will cover the cost of a stander. Once again, a letter of medical necessity, written by your physical therapist or neurologist, is often needed to justify the health benefits to the stander.

96. When should I get a hospital bed?

Hospital beds provide a wealth of benefits to those with trunk and limb weakness. The adjustable height of the bed makes transfers to a walker or wheelchair safer for both the individual and the caretaker than an ordinary bed. The handrails and adjustable head and foot of the bed make repositioning easier for those who cannot turn over easily on their own. The adjustable head of bed is helpful for those with respiratory insufficiency or those who are at risk of aspiration. The adjustable foot of bed is helpful for those who have edema in their legs from long hours in the wheelchair or from cardiac compromise. Finally, the hospital bed can accommodate an alternating pressure mattress for those who are prone to pressure ulcers.

There are three basic styles of hospital beds: manual, semi-electric, or full electric beds. The differences are in how the features are operated. With a manual hospital bed, the foot and head positions and bed height are adjusted manually, typically via a hand crank. Semi-electric hospital beds have a control panel and/or handheld remote that allows the user to adjust the head and foot of the bed, but the bed height is still operated manually. Fully electric hospital beds have a control panel and/or handheld remote that allows the user to control all of the features automatically.

Any one of these benefits may be enough for you to consider getting a hospital bed. Frequently, the decision to buy one of these beds, which cost several thousand dollars, boils down to whether insurance will cover the cost. A hospital bed is generally covered if the individual has a medical condition or pain that requires positioning of the body in ways not feasible with an ordinary bed. Elevation of the head less than 30 degrees does not usually require the use of a hospital bed. Many insurances will only cover a manual or semi-electric bed. The ability to pay the difference to upgrade to a fully electric bed is policy- and provider-specific. Also, some insurance companies may cover the rental of a hospital bed (minus any copays and deductible), but not the purchase of a bed; or, they may apply the rental payments toward the purchase of the bed. As long as insurance is renting or paying for the bed, maintenance costs are typically covered. A letter of medical necessity and a prescription from your provider will be necessary to acquire a hospital bed covered by insurance.

97. What equipment options are there for bathing?

Bathing is such an important aspect of life for hygiene as well as pleasure. However, for those with decreased mobility and their caretakers, the process can be difficult and dangerous. There are several equipment options to assist with bathing.

For those who are ambulatory, grab bars in the shower are essential to provide additional balance and support. Grab bars need to be screwed into studs in the walls for adequate stability. A height-adjustable tub bar to aid in getting in and out of the tub can be easily installed. However, a walk-in shower is safer than having to step over the edge of a bathtub and is a worthwhile investment. Plastic shower chairs or benches make the bathing process less fatiguing and safer. A handheld shower head is helpful in combination with a shower chair. Nonskid mats for the bath or shower reduce the risks of falls.

For those who are nonambulatory and have a bathtub shower, there are bath/shower chairs with a transfer base that goes over the edge of the bathtub. However, these can only be used with a shower curtain and not with shower doors. A single transfer onto the bath/shower chair is needed, and then the individual and chair are slid into the bathtub. For those with a roll-in shower, a shower wheelchair is helpful. One can transfer onto the shower wheelchair in a more convenient location and then wheel into the bathroom where there is often limited room. If there is a small lip at the entrance of the roll-in shower, larger rear wheels on the shower chair will be required. For both the bath/shower chairs with transfer base and the shower wheelchair, there are options for a built-in commode to further decrease the number of transfers. Look for features such as headrest, lateral supports, height adjustable legs, and the ability to tilt the chair. Some of these features can be added to the chair as needed at a later date, and others must be obtained when the chair is ordered.

Your physical and occupational therapists are good resources for finding the best equipment for you for bathing. You will need a letter of medical necessity from your healthcare providers to get insurance coverage for bathing equipment.

98. What help is there for transfers?

As weakness progresses, transferring in and out of bed, wheelchair, toilet, or bath can become difficult and dangerous. There is risk of injury to the individual with MD including dislocation and fracture, as well as risk to the caregiver including back strain and hernia. Specific pieces of equipment can make transfers easier and safer.

If the individual has trunk and upper extremity strength, then a transfer board is helpful. This is an approximately two-foot-long wooden board that goes between objects that are approximately the same height, such as the bed and wheelchair. Advantages to transfer boards include low cost, little space requirement, and ease of use. Disadvantages include the fact that they cannot be used for those who have little trunk and upper extremity strength and that they cause friction from sliding across the board.

An alternative to a transfer board is a Beasy transfer system. The individual is placed on a disc that slides along grooves on the board. This greatly decreases the amount of friction generated. Beasy transfer systems still require trunk and upper extremity strength to operate.

Slings such as that shown in **Figure 14** can be fitted under the individual and with two people can be used to safely lift the individual with MD. Slings come with a variety of supports including head support. A sling can also be connected to a patient lifter (e.g., a Hoyer lift). The lifter can be operated using hydraulic or electric power. An advantage of the hydraulic lift is that it is generally covered by Medicare or insurance, while a disadvantage is that it still requires strength to pump by the caregiver. The power-operated lift is significantly more expensive than the hydraulic lift and is often not covered by Medicare or insurance unless an argument can be made that the caregiver is also disabled. A power-operated lift

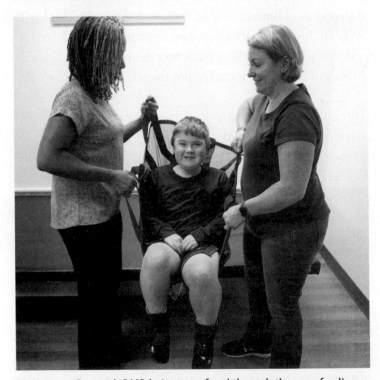

Figure 14 Boy with DMD being transfered through the use of a sling.

significantly decreases the work of lifting and in many cases can be operated by the individual with MD him- or herself once the sling is safely underneath the individual and attached to the lifter. Portable patient lifters that fold and consume less space are also available, but are also not typically covered by insurance.

One of the disadvantages of lifts is that they take up a lot of room and frequently don't fit into small bathrooms. An alternative is a ceiling-mounted track system. In these systems, the sling is connected to hooks hanging from the ceiling that run from room to room. This requires some modifications to the home, including the doorways. Ceiling-mounted track systems are generally not covered by Medicare or insurance. A less expensive option that does not require the same home modifications is a wall-mounted lift. Wall-mounted lifts can be installed over the bed or the toilet and can save space.

There are also different style slings in addition to different style lifts. Slings can be made out of polyester with closed cell foam padding for comfort, an opening for toileting without removing the sling, or fast drying/draining mesh, which enables the sling to also be used for bathing. A U-shaped sling also enables the sling to be easily placed under the individual and removed while in his or her wheelchair. When a sling is left under the individual while sitting in his or her chair, it can cause sliding out of position and also a reduction in the pressure-relieving benefits of the seating components.

What type of transfer system you use depends on your degree of weakness, space, and needs for transfers. Begin with a home OT visit to help make these assessments. Your physician can then provide you with a prescription and letter of medical necessity.

99. What is a loan closet?

The MDA organizes a resource by which eligible individuals can receive gently used equipment free of charge. Equipment is donated to the MDA, and minor repairs are made. This includes wheelchairs, shower chairs, portable ramps, and other durable medical equipment. To be eligible, an individual must be registered with the MDA, have one of the several diagnoses that MDA covers (which includes all MDs), and have a prescription for the equipment item. There is no fee for the service, and individuals can keep the equipment for as long as they have need for it. This is an excellent resource that can truly stretch a limited budget.

100. Can I drive?

Having a physical disability does not exclude a person from obtaining a driver's license. However, there are more steps to the process than for a person who is not disabled. This is due in part, to the need to determine if the person seeking a license is able to safely operate an appropriately modified vehicle. Each state's laws and rules for driving are different, which may mean slight differences in the process based on where one lives.

The first steps for an individual with a disability to obtain a driver's license are taking a written driver's knowledge test and being assessed by a certified driver rehabilitation specialist to determine ability and needed vehicle adaptations and modifications. States may require a formal driver's education training for individuals under a certain age. By age 18, driver's education may not be necessary.

Due to the expense in having a vehicle adapted and modified to accommodate a disabled driver, it may be prudent to have an assessment before proceeding to be certain the individual will meet the requirements. Experienced certified driver rehabilitation specialists are not available in every state. Contact your state Department of Motor Vehicles, accessible vehicle dealer, school guidance department, or area disability rights agency for assistance in locating an individual who can provide the service.

An assessor determines the individual's maturity, judgment, strength, ability, and special needs. This may include ensuring appropriate visual range of motion to see other vehicles from all angles while driving or reaction time and reach in order to safely operate with specialized controls in all conditions. Examples of adaptations include hand controls for an accelerator and brake, joystick control for steering, and push button or touch screen controls for turn signal, lights, and horn. Larger mirrors may be used to compensate for blind spots, although a driver must be aware of traffic operating all around his or her vehicle without restrictions. Modifications may be needed to allow a wheelchair user to enter, transfer to a seat, or remain in his or her personal wheelchair to operate a vehicle. Lowered vehicle floors, raised doors, special wheelchair restraints, automatic doors, and ramps are examples of possible modifications.

The cost of modifying and adapting a van can be expensive, running into the tens of thousands of dollars. Except for special circumstances, the costs will be covered by the individual and his or her family. Resources may be available through the Department of Vocational Rehabilitation (VR) for disabled individuals over age

18 who are seeking employment and/or employment-related training or education. VR is a federal- and state-funded program: https://www.careeronestop.org/ResourcesFor/WorkersWithDisabilities/vocational-rehabilitation.aspx. Programs and resources will vary by state. Some state programs are subject to resource limitations, wait lists, and other impediments that limit their ability to assist students. Disabled students interested in driving can learn more about what resources are available by having their school's guidance department contact a VR case manager. While VR may fund needed modifications and adaptations allowing a disabled individual to drive, families must own or purchase the vehicle.

After passing a written driver's test, a disabled driver has the same requirements to operate an appropriately modified and adapted vehicle under the supervision of a licensed adult and for a specific number of hours, as is required for nondisabled drivers. Depending on the results of their assessment, this may include time with an individual trained in the operation of a vehicle with similar modifications and controls. States may require a second set of vehicle controls (such as an emergency brake pedal) that can be operated by the person supervising the disabled driver in training. After completing the required number of training hours, including nighttime driving, the disabled drivers will schedule a time for a road test with an instructor from the state's Department of Motor Vehicles. Successfully completing a road test allows the individual to operate his or her appropriately adapted vehicle under the similar conditions as required of nondisabled drivers.

Appendix A

Abbreviations

ALT	alanine aminotransferase, a liver enzyme
AST	aspartate aminotransferase, a liver enzyme
BIPAP	bilevel positive airway pressure
BMD	Becker muscular dystrophy, also Bone Mineral Density
CK	creatine kinase
CMD	congenital muscular dystrophy
CPAP	continuous positive airway pressure
DD	distal muscular dystrophy
DM	myotonic muscular dystrophy
DMD	Duchenne muscular dystrophy
EDMD	Emery-Dreifus muscular dystrophy
ECG	electrocardiogram
EMG	electromyography
FEV1	forced expiratory volume measured over 1 second
FSHD	facioscapulohumeral muscular dystrophy
FVC	forced vital capacity
LGMD	limb-girdle muscular dystrophy
MD	muscular dystrophy
MDA	Muscular Dystrophy Association
OPMD	oculopharyngeal muscular dystrophy
OT	occupational therapy
PFT	pulmonary function test
PPMD	Parent Project Muscular Dystrophy
PT	physical therapy
VR	vocational rehabilitation

Appendix B

Foundations That Support Patients and/or Research

Akari Foundation: https://www.theakarifoundation.org/

Brothers Against Duchenne/The Romito Foundation: www.romitofoundation.org/

Charley's Fund: https://charleysfund.org

Coalition Duchenne: http://www.coalitionduchenne.org/

Coalition to Cure Calpain 3: https://curecalpain3.org

Cure CMD: https://curecmd.org

Cure Dale's Duchenne Foundation: http://curedalesduchenne.com/about.html

Cure Duchenne: https://www.cureduchenne.org

Cure LGMD2i: https://curelgmd2i.com

Destroy Duchenne: www.destroyduchenne.org/

Duchenne Family Assistance Program: http://duchennefap.org/index.html

Foundation to Eradicate Duchenne: https://duchennemd.org

Friends of FSH Research: https://www.fshfriends.org

FSHD Society: https://fshdsociety.org

Hope for Gabe: http://www.hopeforgabe.org/

Hope for Gus: https://hopeforgus.org/

Hope for Javier: http://www.hopeforjavier.org/

Jain Foundation: https://www.jain-foundation.org

JB's Keys to DMD: https://www.jbskeys.org/

Jett foundation: https://www.jettfoundation.org

Kurt and Peter Foundation: https://www.kurtpeterfoundation.org/

LGMD2D Foundation: http://lgmd2d.org/

LGMD2iFund: https://www.lgmd2ifund.org

LGMD2L Foundation: https://www.lgmd2l-foundation.org/

Little Hercules Foundation: https://littleherculesfoundation.org

Michael's Cause: https://www.michaelscause.org

Muscular Dystrophy Association: https://www.mda.org

Muscular Dystrophy Family Foundation: https://mdff.org/

Myotonic: https://www.myotonic.org

Parent Project Muscular Dystrophy: https://www.parentprojectmd.org

Pietro's Fight: https://www.pietrosfight.org

Rally for Ryan: https://rallyforryan.org/

Ryan's Hope for a Cure Charitable Foundation: http://www.hopeforryan.com/

Ryan's Quest: https://www.ryansquest.org

Speak Foundation: https://thespeakfoundation.com

StandStrong http://www.standstrongdmd.org/

Suneel's Light: https://www.suneelslight.org/

Team Joseph: https://www.teamjoseph.org/

U.S. Government laws and policies for people with disabilities:
Information on Social Security Disability benefits: https://www.ssa.gov/disability/

Information on the Americans with Disabilities Act (ADA): https://www.ada.gov

Information on the Individuals with Disabilities Education Act (IDEA): https://sites.ed.gov/idea/

Information on Section 504: https://www2.ed.gov/about/offices/list/ocr/504faq.html

GLOSSARY

Glossary

A

Acceptance commitment therapy (ACT): A therapy method based on accepting reality and opening up to unpleasant feelings.

Activities of daily living (ADLs): Activities that everyone participates in day to day, such as dressing, eating, personal hygiene and grooming, and so forth.

Adaptive devices and equipment: Wheelchairs and other devices used to assist disabled persons in mobility or other daily functions.

Allelic disorders: Two or more distinct conditions caused by changes or variants in the same gene. Examples are DMD and BMD.

Ankle foot orthoses (AFOs): A type of brace used in MD that supports the ankle and prevents contracture of the Achilles tendon.

Apnea: The temporary cessation of breathing.

Aquatic therapy: A therapeutic regimen that is conducted in a pool, so that the water can support the body while also providing resistance to work muscles.

Aspiration: Having saliva or food enter the trachea instead of the esophagus. This can lead to choking or pneumonia.

Atelectasis: Collapse of tiny air sacs in the lungs that hold air.

C

Cardiac arrhythmia: An irregular or abnormal heartbeat rhythm.

Cardiologist: A specialist in heart disorders.

Cardiomyopathy: A disorder of the heart muscle.

Cognitive behavioral therapy (CBT): A therapy method aimed to challenge and change distorted thoughts and unhelpful behaviors.

Clinical trial: A research study in human volunteers that is designed to test the safety and/or efficacy of an intervention.

Congenital disease: Disease present at birth.

Contracture: Shortening of muscle and tendon that leads to decreased range of motion.

Creatine kinase (CK): An intracellular enzyme that is elevated in the blood of some forms of MD.

CRISPR: A recently discovered method of genome editing derived from bacteria that targets specific DNA sequences and modifies them.

D

De novo mutation: A genetic alteration that appears for the first time in a family.

Developmental delay: A condition in which a child is not developing or achieving skills according to the expected time frame.

Differentiation: The process in which a stem cell develops into a more specific type of cell, such as a blood or muscle cell.

Double-blinded: A research trial in which neither the volunteer nor the researchers know whether the volunteer was given the actual treatment or the placebo until the end in order to avoid bias.

Dual-energy X-ray absorptiometry: An imaging method that uses X-ray to assess bone density and body composition.

Durable power of attorney for health care: A legal document that identifies another person who can make medical decisions for you if you cannot.

Dysphagia: Difficulty swallowing, as can occur in some MDs such as OPMD, DM, and DMD.

E

Edema: Swelling of a body part, for example in the legs of those sitting in a wheelchair.

Ejection fraction: The percent of blood volume that the ventricles send out to the body. The ejection fraction is an important measure of cardiac function.

Electrocardiogram (ECG): A recording of the electrical activity of the heart that helps identify issues with heart function.

Electromyography (EMG): An electrical recording of muscle activity.

Electrophysiology study: A test of the heart's electrical system in which a wire is inserted through a vein to the heart and electrically stimulates your heart to see how your heart's electrical system responds.

Eligibility criteria: Rules about who can or cannot participate in a clinical trial. These criteria differ from study to study and can include age, gender, specific diagnosis, health history and functional ability.

Executive functions: Cognitive abilities that involve planning and organization as well as self-regulatory skills and self-inhibition.

Exome: The full collection of exons in an individual's genome.

Exon: The protein-coding regions of genes.

F

Fascia: Connective tissue lining of skeletal muscle.

Fat embolism syndrome: An emergency situation in which fat from the bone marrow of a broken bone migrates to other organs including the lungs and brain.

Fibrosis: The condition in which muscle in MD is replaced over time with scar tissue in addition to fat.

Forced expiratory volume measured over 1 second (FEV1): A measure of how much air can be expelled in the first second of exhalation.

Forced vital capacity (FVC): A measure of how much air you can exhale at full capacity, which helps determine the strength of the diaphragm and other respiratory muscles.

G

Gene panel: A genetic testing strategy that reviews multiple genes that are associated with MD.

Gene therapy: The addition, subtraction, or change in genetic material in the cells of an individual who is being treated for a disease.

Genetic Counselor: Genetic counselors provide a critical service to individuals and families considering undergoing genetic testing by helping them identify their risks for certain disorders, investigate family health history, interpret information and determine if testing is needed.

Genome: All the genetic material of an individual.

Genome editing: A procedure that makes permanent changes in the DNA of a living cell in the body.

H

Hand-held dynamometry: A test of muscle strength used to measure the force of muscles.

Hippotherapy: Therapeutic horseback riding.

History: A series of questions the healthcare provider asks to learn more about the patient's background and the disease process, as well as current symptoms or concerns.

I

Implantable cardioverter defibrillator (ICD): An implanted device that continuously monitors heart rhythm and provides high-intensity electrical impulses to restore a normal rhythm if a life-threatening arrhythmia occurs.

Induced pluripotent stem cells (iPSCs): Adult stem cells that have been manipulated in the laboratory to become pluripotent like embryonic stem cells.

Intron: A segment of a gene that does not code for a protein.

L

Liver function tests: A set of laboratory tests that is used to determine the health of the liver. Two of these tests, AST and ALT, are also normally elevated in MD due to the fact that they are produced by muscle as well as liver.

Living will: A legal document that describes your preferences for what treatments should be performed or not performed should you be unable to express them.

M

Muscle biopsy: Removal of a small amount of muscle tissue to gather information for diagnosis or clinical trial purposes.

Mutation: A change in DNA.

Myoglobinuria: Pigmented urine from breakdown of muscle and release of myoglobin into the bloodstream.

Myopathy: Disease of muscle. MD is just one form of myopathy, which is genetic. Others forms of myopathy include inflammatory, toxic, metabolic and endocrine-related myopathies.

N

Neurologist: A doctor who specializes in treating disorder of the nervous system including neuromuscular diseases such as MD.

O

Obsessive–compulsive disorder: A mental health disorder that involves unwanted intrusive thoughts, images, or urges that frequently cause anxiety coupled with a repetitive behavior designed to reduce psychic distress or discomfort.

Obstructive sleep apnea: Interruption of breathing during sleep due to airway obstruction. This is common in people with certain types of MD and obesity.

Oculoplastic surgeon: A surgeon who specializes in ophthalmologic surgery to treat disorders of the eyelids and other regions around the eye.

P

Pacemaker: A battery-operated device implanted under the skin that monitors the heart's electrical activity and supplies electrical impulses when an irregularity occurs.

Paraprofessional: A member of the educational team with at least two years of training, who assists a child with disabilities as part of an IEP or 504 Plan.

Physiatrist: A specialist in physical rehabilitation.

Physical therapy (PT): The treatment of disease, injury, or deformity by physical methods such as massage, heat treatment, and exercise rather than by drugs or surgery.

Placebo: A sham or inactive product that resembles the drug, given to volunteers in a clinical trial as a way of determining a treatment effect.

Pluripotent: Capable of giving rise to several different types of specialized cells.

Polysomnogram: Sleep study in which several body functions are measured including brain activity and oxygen levels, breathing and heartrate.

Port-a-cath: A medical device that is placed under the skin and is connected to a small tube entering the superior vena cava. It is used for the frequent delivery of intravenous medications.

Preclinical studies: Research performed on a new drug prior to entry into human clincial trials.

Prognosis: A prediction of how the disease will progress.

Progressive: A condition that gradually worsens over time.

Protocol: The research plan that describes which individuals are eligible to participate in the trial, what drugs are used and at which dosages, the tests and measures to be performed, and the schedule and duration of the study.

Pseudo-obstruction: An abnormality in the coordinated contraction of the intestines that might be mistaken for bowel obstruction.

Ptosis: Dropping of the upper eyelid.

Pulmonary function test (PFT): Tests performed to assess how well your lungs and related muscles are working to keep oxygen coming in and carbon dioxide going out.

R

Reasonable accommodation: Modifications to a job or work environment that an employer can make to enable an employee with a disability perform essential functions of a job.

Rhabdomyolysis: Massive breakdown of muscle that can occur from exertion, infection or certain anesthetic agents.

S

Satellite cell: An adult stem cell found in skeletal muscle that can replicate and differentiate into new muscle fibers.

Scapular fixation: A surgery in which the scapula is surgically fixed to the rib cage allowing greater range of motion for some individuals with scapular winging.

Scoliosis: Lateral side-to-side curvature of the spine that develops in some MDs due to trunk muscle weakness.

Service animal: As defined by the Americans With Disabilities Act, a dog trained to perform specific functions or behaviors that aid an individual with disabilities.

Side effects: Effects of a treatment that are not the ones intended to treat the disease.

Single gene test: A genetic test that assesses an individual gene associated with the specific type of MD for which there is strong clinical suspicion.

Standard of care: A treatment that is routinely used in day-to-day clinical practice in patients with a specific disease being investigated.

Stem cells: Unspecialized cells that have the ability both to renew themselves and to differentiate into specific types of cells in the body.

Swallowing study: Using X-rays to watch what happens in your mouth, throat, and esophagus as you swallow a special compound visible to the X-ray.

T

Tenotomy: Surgical release of a tendon. Achilles tenotomy may be performed in some with MD to increase the range of motion at the ankle.

Tracheostomy: A surgical opening in the trachea for the purpose of inserting a tube to help a patient breathe.

V

Variant of unknown significance (VUS): A genetic variation in a gene that cannot be definitively determined as causing or not causing disease.

X

X-linked: A gene located on the X chromosome that causes a trait or disorder.

INDEX

Index

Note: Page numbers followed by *f* or *t* indicate material in figures and tables respectively.

A

AAP. *See* American Academy of Pediatrics (AAP)
AAV. *See* adeno-associated virus (AAV)
abnormal gene copy, 31
acceptance commitment therapy (ACT), 140
accommodations
   classroom, 180
   reasonable, 203–206
   requested, 205
   workplace, 207–208
Achilles tendons, 167–168
ACT. *See* acceptance commitment therapy
activities of daily living (ADLs), 10, 52, 212
acupuncture, 157
ADA. *See* Americans with Disabilities Act (ADA)
adaptations, 255
adaptive devices and equipment, 49
adaptive skiing, 218–219
adaptive sports, 218–221
adaptive swimming, 218
adeno-associated virus (AAV), 71
   clinical trials for, 71
   preexisting antibodies to, 72
ADLs. *See* activities of daily living (ADLs)
adolescents, 35

adrenal insufficiency, 136
advance directives, 112–113
aerobic exercise, 46
Affordable Care Act of 2010, 25
AFOs. *See* ankle foot orthoses (AFOs)
airplane travel, tips for, 224–228
alcohol, 132
   affect on muscles, 120–121
   harmful effects of, 120
alcoholic myopathy, 120
allelic disorders, 2
alternative mouse options, 221–222
American Academy of Pediatrics (AAP), 223
Americans with Disabilities Act (ADA), 151, 202–203
anabolic steroids, 59
androgen deficiency, 60
androgen replacement therapy, 60
anesthesia, 103, 173–174
ankle foot orthoses (AFOs), 62–63, 167
antisense oligonucleotide (ASO), 69, 70
   generations of, 70
apnea, 91
aquatic therapy, 49
arrhythmias, 102, 103
ASO. *See* antisense oligonucleotide (ASO)
aspartate aminotransferase (AST), 4, 100
aspiration, 121
AST. *See* aspartate aminotransferase (AST)
atelectasis, 89

attention deficit hyperactivity disorder (ADHD), 193–196
autosomal dominant, 32*f*
autosomal recessive, 33*f*

B

back strain, 251
balanced meals, 118
barium-coated cookie, 121
bathing, 250–251
bathtub shower, 250
battery-operated generator, 107–108
battery-operated recording device, 103
battery-operated ventilator, 226
Beasy transfer system, 251–252
Becker muscular dystrophy (BMD), 2, 4
behavioral therapy, 195
benzodiazepines, 140
bilevel positive airway pressure (BIPAP), 91, 92–94
biventricular pacemaker, 108
blepharoplasty surgery, 172
blood tests, 106
BMD. *See* Becker muscular dystrophy (BMD); bone mineral density (BMD)
BMI. *See* body mass index (BMI)
body mass index (BMI), 119–120
bone density, 60, 117, 131–133
bone fragility, 57
bone mass, 60
bone mineral density (BMD), 130
bracing, 62–63
BRCA genes, 29
buspirone, 140

C

caffeinated beverages, 118
caffeine, 132
calcium, 56
    dietary sources of, 117

cardiac arrhythmias, 102
cardiac resynchronization therapy (CRT), 108–109
cardiomyopathy, 23
cardiopulmonary resuscitation, 113
cardiovascular disease, forms of, 105
cardiovascular risks, 119
CBT. *See* cognitive behavioral therapy (CBT)
ceiling-mounted track systems, 253
children
    mental health, 36
    with muscular dystrophy, 196–199
    sexually active, 35–36
    testing, 36
chronic alcohol consumption, 120
chronic constipation, 125
classroom accommodations, 180
clinical trials, 76–80
    qualify for, 80–81
    risks to participating in, 78–79
Cochrane meta-analysis, 54–55
coenzyme Q10 (CoQ10), 55
cognitive behavioral therapy (CBT), 140
computer mouse, 221–222
congenital disease, 22
congenital muscular dystrophy (CMD), 2
constipation, 125–127
    diagnosis of, 126
    prolonged, 126
    recommendations for treating, 126
    undertreated, 126
continuous positive airway pressure (CPAP), 91, 92–94
contraction, 121
contractures, 48
controller, 221–222
coping, 148
corticosteroids, 56–59, 86, 130
cough, 89–90
CPAP. *See* continuous positive airway pressure (CPAP)

creatine, 54
creatine kinase (CK), 4–5
creatine monohydrate, 55
CRISPR, 73
CRT. *See* cardiac resynchronization
   therapy (CRT)
curriculum, 180
cyberbullying, 223

D

Data and Safety Monitoring Board
   (DSMB), 77
dating and sex, 230–231
day-to-day care, 122
deflazacort, 56
dementia, increased rates of, 207
de novo case, 21
Department of Vocational
   Rehabilitation (VR), 255–256
depression, 140–142, 159–160
developmental delay, 4
DEXA scan, 130–131
dexmethylphenidate, 195
dextroamphetamine, 160, 195
diabetes, 106
diagnosis of MD, 7, 8, 23, 56, 176–177
dietary habits, 125
differentiation, 74
disability, 202
      benefits, 209–210
      information on, 202
      reasonable accommodations to,
         203–206
dislocation, 251
disordered breathing, 91
distal muscular dystrophy (DD), 2
DMD. *See* Duchenne muscular
   dystrophy (DMD)
DMD gene, 69
DNA nucleotides, 22
documentation, 239
domestic flights, 226
dopamine, 195
double-blinded, 78

driver's license, 254–256
dual-chamber pacemaker, 108
Dual-energy X-ray absorptiometry
   (DEXA), 130
Duchenne muscular dystrophy
   (DMD), 2, 4, 15*f*, 16, 35, 57,
   59–60, 64, 68, 71
      carriers of, 23
      dystrophin, 68, 68*f*
      setting of, 58
      treatment of, 57
durable power of attorney for health
   care, 112
dysphagia, 121
dystrophin, 68

E

echocardiogram, 103–105, 105*f*
edema, 242
educational impact, 178
ejection fraction, 104
electrical wave, 102–103
electrocardiogram (ECG), 102–103,
   110
electromyography (EMG), 6
electrophysiology study, 107
elevated cholesterol, 106
eligibility criteria, 80–81
emergency department (ED), 98–100
Emery-Dreifus muscular dystrophy
   (EDMD), 2
employer, 202–203
employment
      agencies, 212
      benefits of, 202, 203, 207
      privileges of, 203
endorphins, 157
endoscopic approach, 123
energy conservation therapy, 160
energy metabolism, 55
enzymes, 100
epigallocatechin gallate (EGCG), 56
ES. *See* exome sequencing (ES)
esophagus, 121–122

event monitors, 103

executive dysfunction, medications for, 149

executive functions, 147–149

exercises, 46–47, 132
    to combat atrophy of muscles, 47

exome, 27

exome sequencing (ES), 26
    challenge with, 28

exons, 27
    skipping, 68–70, 68f

extreme limitation, 209

F

facioscapulohumeral muscular dystrophy (FSHD), 30, 170f

Family and Medical Leave Act (FMLA), 210–212

family stress, 36–37

fascia, 82

fat embolism syndrome, 99, 136

fatigue, 159–161, 206

fatty fish, 134

faulty gene, 38–39

federal funding, 180

feedings, 123

fiber consumption, 118

fibrosis, 2

504 Plan, 178–181

FMLA. See Family and Medical Leave Act (FMLA)

forced expiratory volume measured over 1 second (FEV1), 88

forced vital capacity (FVC), 88

fractures, 60, 135–137, 251

front wheel drive, 241

full electric beds, 249

FVC. See forced vital capacity (FVC)

G

gamma glutamyl transferase (GGT) test, 100

gastrostomy tube, 122–125, 125f

gene panel, 26

gene therapy, 70–72
    effectiveness of, 72

genetic counselors, 36, 40–41

Genetic Information Nondiscrimination Act (GINA), 25

genetics
    disease, 20–22
    exome sequencing (ES), 27–29
    testing, 22–26

genetic testing, 35–36
    cost of, 26

genome, 27
    editing, 73–74

GGT test. See gamma glutamyl transferase (GGT) test

glucose tolerance tests, 106

Gower's maneuver, 4

green tea extract, 55–56

H

handheld dynamometry, 14–15

handrails, 248

healthcare professionals, 239

healthcare providers, 37

healthy weight, 118–120

heart
    attack, 105–106
    pump function of, 102
    steps to protect, 105–107
    valves, structure and function of, 104

hemoglobin A1C, 106

hernia, 251

high blood pressure, 105

hippotherapy, 218, 220

history, 14

hospital beds, 248–249
    styles of, 249

human embryonic stem cells, 74

human volunteers, 76

hydration, 123

hydraulic lift, 252
hypoxia, 91

I

ICD. *See* implantable cardioverter
    defibrillator (ICD)
IEP. *See* Individual Education
    Plan (IEP)
immobility, 117, 135
immunosuppression, 86
implantable cardioverter defibrillator
    (ICD), 109, 110–112
    battery, 111
    functions, 111
    implantation of, 111
impurities, 56
incidental findings, 29
Individual Education Plan (IEP),
    176, 178–181
individual needs, 190, 237
Individuals with Disabilities
    Education Act (IDEA), 178
induced pluripotent stem cells
    (iPSCs), 75
influenza vaccines, 86–87
inhaled anesthetic agents, 173
Institutional Review Board (IRB), 76
intramuscularly (IM), 57
intravenous bisphosphonates, 136
introns, 68, 68*f*
invasive mechanical ventilation, 97
    advantages and disadvantages of,
        96–98
in vitro fertilization, 74
IRB. *See* Institutional Review Board
    (IRB)

J

job performance, 202, 205

L

L-arginine, 55
L-citrulline, 55

lifts, 252
    disadvantages of, 253
limb-girdle muscular dystrophy
    (LGMD), 2
live attenuated vaccines, 87
liver function tests, 4, 100
living wills, 112
loan closet, 254

M

macronutrients, 117
manifesting carrier, 21
manual hospital bed, 249
manual muscle testing, 14
marked limitation, 209
massage therapy, 157
MD. *See* muscular
    dystrophy (MD)
media, 222–224
    devices, 223
Medicaid, 213
medical necessity, 49
medical therapies, 126
Medicare, 213, 248, 252
medications, 132–133, 160, 195
mental ailment, 209
mental health therapy, 140
metformin, 55
methylphenidate, 194, 195
midline back pain, 135
mid wheel drive wheelchair, 241
modafinil, 160
mood disturbance, 57
Multiple Ascending Dose (MAD)
    trial, 77
muscles, 44–45*f*
    atrophy of, 47
    biopsy, 81–83
    damage to, 47
    disorder, diagnosis of, 7
    fibers, 74–75
    involvement, 7
    supplements for, 54–56
    weakness of, 45–46

muscular dystrophy (MD), 2–3,
    36–40, 119–121
    autosomal recessive, 20–21, 31
    carriers of, 30–34
    causes of, 44
    clinical trials for, 23, 71
    conversations about, 38
    creatine in, 54–55
    diagnosis of, 6–9
    dominant, 20–21
    end stage of, 44
    exon-skipping drug for, 69
    families affected with, 16–18
    family history of, 24
    genes, 7, 29
    genetic types of, 28
    individuals with, 117, 210, 230
    inheritance of, 20, 22
    initial signs of, 3–6
    management of, 47–48
    medical care, 9–13
    neurology appointment, 13–16
    pregnancy with, 231–233
    progressive, 24, 206
    reasonable accommodations,
        203–206
    recessive, 21
    risk of developing, 23
    symptoms of, 21, 125–127
    types of, 31
    use of supplements in, 54
    weakness in, 45
    working with progressive, 206–209
    X-linked, 21
Muscular Dystrophy Association
    (MDA), 11, 176–177, 254
musculoskeletal pain, 156
myoglobinuria, 47
myopathy, 120–121
    alcoholic, 120

N

needle muscle biopsies, 82–83
neurologist, 6, 10, 13–16

neuromuscular physician, 159
neuropsychological evaluation,
    142–144
nondisabled drivers, 256
noninvasive mechanical ventilation,
    advantages and disadvantages of,
    94–95
nonsteroidal anti-inflammatory
    medications (NSAIDs), 156–157
norepinephrine, 195
nutrition, 116–118, 123, 131–132
nutritional recommendations,
    116–118

O

obsessive–compulsive disorder (OCD),
    150–151
    common symptoms of, 150
obstructive sleep apnea (OSA),
    92, 159
occupational therapist (OT), 10,
    52, 53f
occupational therapy (OT), 52–54,
    180
oculopharyngeal muscular dystrophy
    (OPMD), 2, 28
oculoplastic surgeon, 172–173
one-on-one paraprofessional, 186
online predators, 223
online socialization, 222–224
Open Label Extension (OLE)
    studies, 77
opioids, 157
optimal muscle health, 118
osteoporosis, 60
overweight, 119
oxandrolone, 59–60
oxidative stress, 55

P

pacemakers, 107–111
    battery, 108
    information on, 110

insertion, 108
types of, 108
pain, 156–159, 161
sources of, 156
types and causes of, 156
palliative care, 162–163
referral to, 163
paraprofessional, 185–186
parasports, 218–221
Parent Project Muscular Dystrophy
(PPMD), 64, 176, 177
Parent Training in Behavior
Management (PTBM), 194
pathogenic variant, 28
PCA. See personal care attendant or
assistant (PCA)
PEG. See percutaneous endoscopic
gastrostomy (PEG)
percutaneous endoscopic gastrostomy
(PEG), 123
perinatal stem cells, 75
personal care attendant or assistant
(PCA), 212
personal care attendant support,
212–215
PFT. See pulmonary function test
(PFT)
physiatrist, 10
physical ailment, 209
physical therapist (PT), 10
physical therapy (PT), 47–51
placebo, 78
plastic shower chairs, 250
pluripotent, 74
pneumococcus, 86
pneumonia, 86
Pneumovax 23 (PPSV23), 87
polysomnogram, 91
portable patient lifters, 253
port-a-cath, 70
postanesthesia care unit, 174
postmarketing surveillance, 78
postoperative use of sedatives and
opiates, 174
power anterior tilt, 243

power elevating leg
rests, 242
power mobility device, 236
power recline, 242
power scooters, 236–237
advantages and disadvantages of,
236–237
power seat elevate, 242–243
power seating, features, 241–244
power soccer, 218
power standing, 243–244
power tilt, 241–242
power wheelchair, 237–240
advantages and disadvantages
of, 238
controls, 244
postural supports, 245–246
PPMD. See Parent Project
Muscular Dystrophy (PPMD)
preclinical studies, 76
prediabetes, 106
prednisolone, 56
prednisone, 56
pregnancy, 231–233
prevent clogging, 123
Prevnar 13 (PCV13), 86–87
primary care provider, 159
private health, 207
private school, 181–184
prognosis, 7
progression, rates of, 45
progressive disorder of muscle, 2
proper micronutrients, 117
proper nutrition, 124
protein, 117
protocol of clinical trials, 76
pseudo-obstruction, 99
PTBM. See Parent Training in
Behavior Management
(PTBM)
ptosis, 172
repair, 172–173
public school, 181–184
pulmonary function test (PFT),
87–88

Q

quality of life, 156, 167
  focus on, 163
  suffering and improvement of, 162

R

rate of progression, 15
reading, and writing, 190–193
rear wheel drive wheelchair, 241
reasonable accommodations, 203–206
  to disabilities, 203–206
rehabilitation facility, 167
rehabilitative physical therapy, 170
requested accommodation, 205
retinal dystrophy, gene therapies
  for, 71
retirement benefits, 207
rhabdomyolysis, 86, 173

S

sailing, 219, 219f
satellite cells, 74
  transplantation of, 74
scapular fixation, 169–172
  risks to, 170
schools, 186–187
  reasonable accommodations,
    186–189
scoliosis, 166
  surgery, 166–167
secondary findings, 29
selective serotonin reuptake inhibitors
  (SSRIs), 140
self-advocacy, 226
self-reflection, 205
semi-electric hospital bed, 249
serial casting, 169
serotonin and norepinephrine
  reuptake inhibitors (SNRIs), 140
service animal, 151–154
service dogs, 151, 152f, 153
service plan, 182

sex, dating and, 230–231
sexting, 223
side effects of drug, 77
Single Ascending Dose (SAD)
  trial, 77
single-chamber leadless pacemakers, 108
single-chamber pacemaker, 108
single gene test, 25
sip and puff ventilation, 95–96, 96f
sleep-disordered breathing, 91
sleep study, 91
slings, 252, 252f, 253
smoking, 132
social history, 14
social media, 222–224
Social Security Administration
  (SSA), 207, 209
    qualifications for disability, 210
Social Security Disability Insurance
  (SSDI), 209–210
special education services, 179
spirometry, 87–88
SSA. See Social Security
  Administration (SSA)
SSDI. See Social Security Disability
  Insurance (SSDI)
stamina, strength and, 161–162
standard of care, 78
stander, 246–248, 247f
stem cells, 74–76
stem cell therapy, 75–76
stimulant laxatives, 127
strength, and stamina, 161–162
Streptococcus pneumoniae, 86
stretching, 157
  general rules regarding, 63–65
succinylcholine, 173
support group, 144–147
swallowing study, 121–122

T

TCAs. See tricyclic antidepressants
  (TCAs)
technology, 222

tendon, 168–169
  releases, 167–169
tenotomy, 168
testosterone, 59–62
tobacco use, 106–107
tracheostomy, 97
transcutaneous electrical nerve
  stimulation (TENS), 157
transfer board, 251–252
transfers, 251–253
transition planning, 196
Transition Toolkit for DMD, 196
travel, tips for, 224–228
tricyclic antidepressants (TCAs), 140
tube feeds, 123

U

ubiquinone, 55
unemployment, risks of, 207

V

variant of unknown significance
  (VUS), 28–29
vehicle controls, 256
ventilatory support, 90–92

vertebral fractures, 135–136
video games, 222–224
viruses, 71
vitamin D, 56, 134–135
volunteers, 76–77
VUS. *See* variant of unknown
  significance (VUS)

W

weight, 132
wheelchair, 49, 52, 95, 96, 137, 152,
  218, 225, 236
  features, 240–241
Wheelchair Assistance Dogs, 152,
  152*f*
wheelchair tennis, 218
Whole Exome Sequencing
  (WES), 27
work environment, 205
workplace, accommodations, 207–208
writing, 191

X

X-linked disorder, 31
X-linked recessive, 34*f*

Acknowledgments

This book has benefited from the advice of many healthcare professionals, patients, and families. I learn from my patients every day, and I am immensely grateful for all that they have taught me about muscular dystrophy and life. I would like to thank Julie Cohen for her input on genetics, James Poysky for his input on psychological issues, Charlie Wiener and Rebecca Dezube for their input on pulmonary issues, Shree Pandya and Nikia Stinson for their input on physical therapy, Susan Schiaffino for her input on occupational therapy and equipment, Janet Crane for her input on endocrinology, Andrea Heyman for her input on nutrition, Brian Denger for his input on driving, Andreas Barth for his input on cardiology, Kent Williams for his input on gastroenterology, Gail Geller for her input on palliative care, Shannath Merbs for her input on ptosis repair, Paul Sponseller for his input on scoliosis surgery, Kiley Morgart for school and work-related issues, Rachel Morgan and Linda Prudente for photography, Arjun Ramesh for illustrations, and Jordan Reidenberg, Nicolas Raymond, Nikia Stinson, Ryan Bianco, Chrissy Bianco, Jason Vogel, Lilleen Walters, Collin Walters, Courtney Fiorini, Deanna Johnson, Tayjus Surampudi, James Shrybman, Carly Scrivener, Jessica Ryley Hammond, and Colin Smith for serving as models.

I would particularly like to thank the four individuals, Tayjus Surampudi, Vicky Bhalla Singh, Lilleen Walters, and Colin Smith who shared their own experiences with MD in such open and insightful ways. They have made this book relevant and relatable.

I would like to thank Sarepta Therapeutics for sponsoring the production of this book.

Finally, I would like to thank my sister, Krystn Wagner, for suggesting that I write this book, for helpful edits, and for a lifetime of support.

Patient Commentary Biographies

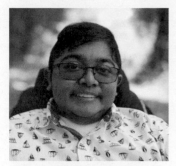

Tayjus Surampudi is a 24-year-old living with DMD, originally from New Jersey. Despite having DMD, Tayjus has never let it get in his way. He graduated from Harvard in 2018, where he studied Government and Health Policy. He has also served as a patient advocate for DMD and rare diseases, having spoken at several biotech and pharmaceutical companies about his experience. Tayjus hopes to continue his patient advocacy and ensure that the voices of people with MD do not go unheard. He currently lives in the San Francisco Bay Area where he works for Google.

Courtesy of Levi Gershkowitz, Living in the Light - www.FromPatientToPerson.com; Courtesy of Tayjus Surampudi

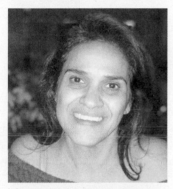

Vicky Bhalla Singh was born in London, grew up in New York, has lived and worked on four continents and currently resides in Potomac, MD. She has two children, her son, Saij, who is off to college next year and her daughter, Kaveen, a recent Master's graduate. In 2010, Vicky ran the NYC marathon to create awareness of DMD and to raise funds to find a cure. She later started a 501-c3, charitable organization, Stand Strong, which has raised close to $1M to expedite treatment paths to help Saij and all other boys living with DMD. Vicky enjoys being outdoors, cooking, reading, and practicing yoga.

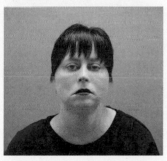

Lilleen C. Walters was born in San Diego, CA, in 1968, the youngest of six children. A military brat, Lilleen lived around the world and graduated high school in Naples, Italy. Lilleen and her husband Gary have been happily married for 30 years. They have two grown children, Collin and Catherine. After graduating from Georgia Military Academy in 1992, Lilleen worked for the Department of Defense. Presently, she is a business owner of a personal finance company. Lilleen was diagnosed with FSHD when she was 15 years old. She continues to be active and involved helping others diagnosed with MD.

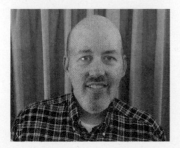

Colin Smith was born and raised in Vermont. He has lived in many parts of the United States including New England, the Pacific Northwest, and California. In 2000 when he was 26, Colin was diganosed with Myotonic muscular dystrophy as was his father and younger sister. He experienced isolation and depression. In 2011, after a 10-year hiatus, Colin rediscovered his passion for sailing. Adaptive sailing and racing have become a major part of his life. Currently Colin lives in Middlebury, Vermont, taking life one day at a time and striving to not let his disability define him.